Medifocus Guidebook on:

Parkinson's Disease

Last Update: 05 July 2018

Medifocus.com, Inc.

6810 Park Heights Ave.
Suite C5
Baltimore, MD 21215

www.medifocus.com

(800) 965-3002

MediFocus Guide #NR013

How To Use This Medifocus Guidebook

Before you start to review your *Guidebook*, it would be helpful to familiarize yourself with the organization and content of the information that is included in the Guidebook. Your *MediFocus Guidebook* is organized into the following five major sections.

- **Section 1: Background Information** - This section provides detailed information about the organization and content of the *Guidebook* including tips and suggestions for conducting additional research about the condition.
- **Section 2: The Intelligent Patient Overview** - This section is a comprehensive overview of the condition and includes important information about the cause of the disease, signs and symptoms, how the condition is diagnosed, the treatment options, quality of life issues, and questions to ask your doctor.
- **Section 3: Guide to the Medical Literature** - This section opens the door to the latest cutting-edge research and clinical advances recently published in leading medical journals. It consists of an extensive, focused selection of journal article references with links to the PubMed® abstracts (summaries) of the articles. PubMed® is the U.S. National Library of Medicine's database of references and abstracts from more than 4,500 medical and scientific articles published worldwide.
- **Section 4: Centers of Research** - This section is a unique directory of doctors, researchers, hospitals, medical centers, and research institutions with specialized interest and, in many cases, clinical expertise in the management of patients with the condition. You can use the "Centers of Research" directory to contact, consults, or network with leading experts in the field and to locate a hospital or medical center that can help you.
- **Section 5: Tips for Finding and Choosing a Doctor** - This section of your *Guidebook* offers important tips for how to find physicians as well as suggestions for how to make informed choices about choosing a doctor who is right for you.
- **Section 6: Directory of Organizations** - This section of your *Guidebook* is a directory of select disease organizations and support groups that are in the business of helping patients and their families by providing access to information, resources, and services. Many of these organizations can answer your questions, enable you to network with other patients, and help you find a doctor in your geographical area who specializes in managing your condition.

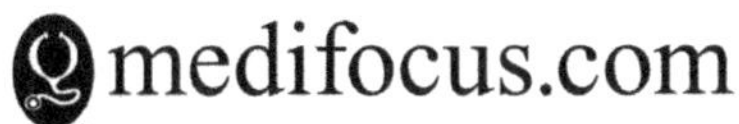

Disclaimer

Medifocus.com, Inc. serves only as a clearinghouse for medical health information and does not directly or indirectly practice medicine. Any information provided by *Medifocus.com, Inc.* is intended solely for educating our clients and should not be construed as medical advice or guidance, which should always be obtained from a licensed physician or other health-care professional. As such, the client assumes full responsibility for the appropriate use of the medical and health information contained in the Guidebook and agrees to hold *Medifocus.com, Inc.* and any of its third-party providers harmless from any and all claims or actions arising from the clients' use or reliance on the information contained in this Guidebook. Although *Medifocus.com, Inc.* makes every reasonable attempt to conduct a thorough search of the published medical literature, the possibility always exists that some significant articles may be missed.

Copyright

Table of Contents

1 - Background Information

Introduction

Chronic or life-threatening illnesses can have a devastating impact on both the patient and the family. In today's new world of medicine, many consumers have come to realize that they are the ones who are primarily responsible for their own health care as well as for the health care of their loved ones.

When facing a chronic or life-threatening illness, you need to become an educated consumer in order to make an informed health care decision. Essentially that means finding out everything about the illness - the treatment options, the doctors, and the hospitals - so that you can become an educated health care consumer and make the tough decisions. In the past, consumers would go to a library and read everything available about a particular illness or medical condition. In today's world, many turn to the Internet for their medical information needs.

The first sites visited are usually the well known health "portals" or disease organizations and support groups which contain a general overview of the condition for the layperson. That's a good start but soon all of the basic information is exhausted and the need for more advanced information still exists. What are the latest "cutting-edge" treatment options? What are the results of the most up-to-date clinical trials? Who are the most notable experts? Where are the top-ranked medical institutions and hospitals?

The best source for authoritative medical information in the United States is the National Library of Medicine's medical database called PubMed®, that indexes citations and abstracts (brief summaries) of over 7 million articles from more than 3,800 medical journals published worldwide. PubMed® was developed for medical professionals and is the primary source utilized by health care providers for keeping up with the latest advances in clinical medicine.

A typical PubMed® search for a specific disease or condition, however, usually retrieves hundreds or even thousands of "hits" of journal article citations. That's an avalanche of information that needs to be evaluated and transformed into truly useful knowledge. What are the most relevant journal articles? Which ones apply to your specific situation? Which articles are considered to be the most authoritative - the ones your physician would rely on in making clinical decisions? This is where *Medifocus.com* provides an effective solution.

Medifocus.com has developed an extensive library of *MediFocus Guidebooks* covering a wide spectrum of chronic and life threatening diseases. Each *MediFocus Guidebook* is a high quality, up- to-date digest of "professional-level" medical information consisting of the most relevant citations and abstracts of journal articles published in authoritative, trustworthy medical journals. This information represents the latest advances known to modern medicine for the treatment and management of the condition, including published results from clinical trials. Each *Guidebook* also includes a valuable index of leading authors and medical institutions as well as a directory of disease organizations and support groups. *MediFocus Guidebooks* are reviewed, revised and updated every 4-months to ensure that you receive the latest and most up-to-date information about the specific condition.

About Your MediFocus Guidebook

Introduction

Your *MediFocus Guidebook* is a valuable resource that represents a comprehensive synthesis of the most up-to-date, advanced medical information published about the condition in well-respected, trustworthy medical journals. It is the same type of professional-level information used by physicians and other health-care professionals to keep abreast of the latest developments in biomedical research and clinical medicine. The *Guidebook* is intended for patients who have a need for more advanced, in-depth medical information than is generally available to consumers from a variety of other resources. The primary goal of a *MediFocus Guidebook* is to educate patients and their families about their treatment options so that they can make informed health-care decisions and become active participants in the medical decision making process.

The *Guidebook* production process involves a team of experienced medical research professionals with vast experience in researching the published medical literature. This team approach to the development and production of the *MediFocus Guidebooks* is designed to ensure the accuracy, completeness, and clinical relevance of the information. The *Guidebook* is intended to serve as a basis for a more meaningful discussion between patients and their health-care providers in a joint effort to seek the most appropriate course of treatment for the disease.

Guidebook Organization and Content

Section 1 - Background Information

This section provides detailed information about the organization and content of the *Guidebook* including tips and suggestions for conducting additional research about the condition.

Section 2 - The Intelligent Patient Overview

This section of your *MediFocus Guidebook* represents a detailed overview of the disease or condition specifically written from the patient's perspective. It is designed to satisfy the basic informational needs of consumers and their families who are confronted with the illness and are facing difficult choices. Important aspects which are addressed in "The Intelligent Patient" section include:

- The etiology or cause of the disease
- Signs and symptoms
- How the condition is diagnosed

- The current standard of care for the disease
- Treatment options
- New developments
- Important questions to ask your health care provider

Section 3 - Guide to the Medical Literature

This is a roadmap to important and up-to-date medical literature published about the condition from authoritative, trustworthy medical journals. This is the same information that is used by physicians and researchers to keep up with the latest developments and breakthroughs in clinical medicine and biomedical research. A broad spectrum of articles is included in each *MediFocus Guidebook* to provide information about standard treatments, treatment options, new clinical developments, and advances in research. To facilitate your review and analysis of this information, the articles are grouped by specific categories. A typical *MediFocus Guidebook* usually contains one or more of the following article groupings:

- *Review Articles:* Articles included in this category are broad in scope and are intended to provide the reader with a detailed overview of the condition including such important aspects as its cause, diagnosis, treatment, and new advances.

- *General Interest Articles:* These articles are broad in scope and contain supplementary information about the condition that may be of interest to select groups of patients.

- *Drug Therapy:* Articles that provide information about the effectiveness of specific drugs or other biological agents for the treatment of the condition.

- *Surgical Therapy:* Articles that provide information about specific surgical treatments for the condition.

- *Clinical Trials:* Articles in this category summarize studies which compare the safety and efficacy of a new, experimental treatment modality to currently available standard treatments for the condition. In many cases, clinical trials represent the latest advances in the field and may be considered as being on the "cutting edge" of medicine. Some of these experimental treatments may have already been incorporated into clinical practice.

The following information is provided for each of the articles referenced in this section of your *MediFocus Guidebook:*

- Article title

- Author Name(s)
- Institution where the study was done
- Journal reference (Volume, page numbers, year of publication)
- Link to Abstract (brief summary of the actual article)

Linking to Abstracts: Most of the medical journal articles referenced in this section of your *MediFocus Guidebook* include an abstract (brief summary of the actual article) that can be accessed online via the National Library of Medicine's PubMed® database. You can easily access the individual abstracts online via PubMed® from the "electronic" format of your *MediFocus Guidebook* by clicking on the corresponding URL address that is provided for each cited article. If you purchased a printed copy of a *MediFocus Guidebook*, you can still access the article abstracts online by entering the individual URL address for a particular article into your web browser.

Section 4 - Centers of Research

We've compiled a unique directory of doctors, researchers, medical centers, and research institutions with specialized research interest, and in many cases, clinical expertise in the management of the specific medical condition. The "Centers of Research" directory is a valuable resource for quickly identifying and locating leading medical authorities and medical institutions within the United States and other countries that are considered to be at the forefront in clinical research and treatment of the condition.

Inclusion of the names of specific doctors, researchers, hospitals, medical centers, or research institutions in this *Guidebook* does not imply endorsement by Medifocus.com, Inc. or any of its affiliates. Consumers are encouraged to conduct additional research to identify health-care professionals, hospitals, and medical institutions with expertise in providing specific medical advice, guidance, and treatment for this condition.

Section 5 - Tips on Finding and Choosing a Doctor

One of the most important decisions confronting patients who have been diagnosed with a serious medical condition is finding and choosing a qualified physician who will deliver high-level, quality medical care in accordance with curently accepted guidelines and standards of care. Finding the "best" doctor to manage your condition, however, can be a frustrating and time-consuming experience unless you know what you are looking for and how to go about finding it. This section of your Guidebook offers important tips for how to find physicians as well as suggestions for how to make informed choices about choosing a doctor who is right for you.

Section 6 - Directory of Organizations

This section of your *Guidebook* is a directory of select disease organizations and support groups that are in the business of helping patients and their families by providing access to information, resources, and services. Many of these organizations can answer your questions, enable you to network with other patients, and help you find a doctor in your geographical area who specializes in managing your condition.

Ordering Full-Text Articles

After reviewing your *MediFocus Guidebook*, you may wish to order the full-text copy of some of the journal article citations that are referenced in the *Guidebook*. There are several options available for obtaining full-text copies of journal articles, however, with the exception of obtaining the article yourself by visiting a nearby medical library, most involve a fee to cover the costs of photocopying, delivering, and paying the copyright royalty fees set by the individual publishers of medical journals.

This section of your *MediFocus Guidebook* provides some basic information about how you can go about obtaining full-text copies of journal articles from various fee-based document delivery resources.

Commercial Document Delivery Services

There are numerous commercial document delivery companies that provide full-text photocopying and delivery services to the general public. The costs may vary from company to company so it is worth your while to carefully shop-around and compare prices. Some of these commercial document delivery services enable you to order articles directly online from the company's web site. You can locate companies that provide document delivery services by typing the key words "document delivery" into any major Internet search engine.

National Library of Medicine's "Loansome Doc" Document Retrieval Services

The National Library of Medicine (NLM), located in Bethesda, Maryland, offers full-text photocopying and delivery of journal articles through its on-line service known as "Loansome Doc". To learn more about how you can order articles using "Loansome Doc", please visit the NLM web site at:
http://www.nlm.nih.gov/pubs/factsheets/loansome_doc.html

Participating "Loansome Doc" Libraries: United States

In the United States there are approximately 250 medical libraries that participate in the National Library of Medicine's "Loansome Doc" document retrieval and delivery services for the general public. Please note that each participating library sets its own policies and charges for providing document retrieval services. To order full-text copies of articles, simply contact a participating "Loansome Doc" medical library in your geographical area and ask to speak with one of the reference librarians. They can answer all of your questions including fees, delivery options, and turn-around time.

Here is how to find a participating "Loansome Doc" library in the U.S. that provides article retrieval services for the general public:

- **United States** - Contact a Regional Medical Library at 1-800-338-7657 (Monday - Friday; 8:30 AM - 5:30 PM). They will provide information about libraries in your area with which you may establish an account for the "Loansome Doc" service.

- **Canada** - Contact the Canada Institute for Scientific and Technical Information (CISTI) at 1-800-668-1222 for information about libraries in your area.

International MEDLARS Centers

If you reside outside the United States, you can obtain copies of medical journal articles through one of several participating International Medical Literature Analysis and Retrieval Systems (MEDLARS) Centers that provide "Loansome Doc" services in over 20 major countries. International MEDLARS Centers can be found in some of these countries: Australia, Canada, China, Egypt, France, Germany, Hong Kong, India, Israel, Italy, Japan, Korea, Kuwait, Mexico, Norway, Russia, South Africa, Sweden, and the United Kingdom. A complete listing of International MEDLARS Centers, including locations and telephone contact information can be viewed at:
http://www.nlm.nih.gov/pubs/factsheets/intlmedlars.html

NOTES

Use this page for taking notes as you review your Guidebook

2 - The Intelligent Patient Overview

PARKINSON'S DISEASE

Introduction to Parkinson's Disease

Parkinson's disease (PD) is a progressive, neurodegenerative disorder that affects movement, muscle control, and balance, as well as numerous other motor and non-motor functions. It is part of a group of conditions known as *motor systems disorders*. Parkinson's disease was named for James Parkinson, a general practitioner in London who first described the symptoms of the disease during the 19th century. Symptoms describing Parkinson's disease are mentioned in the writings of medicine in India dating back to 5,000 BCE, as well as in Chinese writings dating back approximately 2,500 years. Parkinson's disease is the most common movement disorder, and the second most common neurodegenerative disorder, following Alzheimer's disease.

The underlying disease process of Parkinson's disease involves the death of dopamine-producing cells and the subsequent reduction of available dopamine in the brain which affects motor function. The hallmark symptoms of Parkinson's disease (PD) are asymmetric (one side of the body) tremors at rest, rigidity (muscle stiffness), *bradykinesia* (slowness in movement), and impairment of gait and posture (walking and standing erect). There is currently no cure for Parkinson's disease; it is always chronic and progressive, meaning that the symptoms always exist and always worsen over time. The rate of progression varies from person to person, as does the intensity of the symptoms. While walking, balance, muscle control and coordination are affected, Parkinson's disease itself is not a fatal disease and many people live with Parkinson's into their older years. Mortality of individuals with PD is usually attributable to secondary complications, such as pneumonia or fall-related injuries.

There are three types of Parkinson's disease and they are grouped by age of onset:

- *Adult-Onset Parkinson's Disease* - This is the most common type of Parkinson's disease. The average age of onset is approximately 60 years old. The incidence of Adult-Onset PD rises noticeably as people advance in age (70's and 80's).

- *Young-Onset Parkinson's Disease* - The age of onset is between 21-40 years old. Though the incidence of Young-Onset Parkinson's disease is very high in Japan (approximately 40% of cases diagnosed with Parkinson's disease in Japan), it is still relatively uncommon in the U.S., with estimates ranging from 5-10% of PD cases diagnosed.

- *Juvenile Parkinson's Disease* - The age of onset is before the age of 21. The incidence of Juvenile Parkinson's disease is very low.

There are hereditary forms of PD that affect up to 15% of individuals with Parkinson's disease and are usually associated with Juvenile or Adult-Onset PD.

Parkinson's disease significantly impairs quality of life, not only for individuals with PD but for their families as well, and especially for their primary caregivers. It is therefore important for caregivers and family members to educate themselves and become familiar with the course of Parkinson's disease and the progression of symptoms so that they can be actively involved in communication with health care providers and in understanding all decisions regarding treatment.

Incidence of Parkinson's Disease

According to the American Parkinson's Disease Association (APDA), there are approximately 1.5 million people in the U.S. who suffer from Parkinson's disease - approximately 1-2% of people over the age of 60, and 3-5% of the population over age 85. The incidence of PD ranges from 8.6 - 19 per 100,000 people. Approximately 50,000 new cases are diagnosed in the U.S. annually. That number is expected to rise as the general population in the U.S. ages. All races and ethnic groups are affected.

The incidence of Parkinson's disease among males and females is generally equally distributed when onset of disease is before the age of 60. When onset is past 60 years of age, most studies report a higher incidence in males.

Pathophysiology of Parkinson's Disease

Increasing evidence suggests that Parkinson's disease is a multi-system brain disease in which various neurotransmitter systems are affected, including those controlling voluntary movement.

Deep in the brain, below the cerebral cortex, there are interconnected areas of grey matter collectively known as the *basal ganglia* (literally "basement structures"). These structures include the *caudate nucleus*, *putamen*, and *globus pallidum internus* (GPi) which are involved in controlling voluntary movement. Next to the basal ganglia are a cluster of nerve cells called the *substantia nigra* which produce *dopamine*, an essential neurotransmitter that is responsible for transmitting electrical signals between nerve cells to regulate movement. The substantia nigra sends out fibers to the *corpus striatum* (bands of tissue in the caudate nucleus and putamen) where the dopamine is released. The transmission of dopamine and its release into the corpus striatum is necessary for smooth, coordinated muscle movement.

Parkinson's disease occurs when there is a disruption of dopamine production, which leads to impaired neurotransmission (communication between brain cells) in the basal ganglia. As the nerve cells in the brain that make dopamine are destroyed, the reduced levels of dopamine cause the nerve cells to fire out of control, resulting in a loss of smooth, controlled muscle activity. The death of dopamine-producing cells in the substantia nigra leads to reduced levels of dopamine reaching the corpus striatum, and this is the primary pathology in Parkinson's disease. By the time symptoms develop, there is at least a 60% loss of dopamine-producing cells in the substantia nigra, and an 80-90% loss of dopamine in the corpus striatum.

Parkinson's disease is also characterized by the presence of *Lewy bodies*, abnormal structures that are found in the nerve cells of the substantia nigra as well as in other secondary locations. Lewy bodies are strongly correlated with neurodegeneration and are considered a diagnostic hallmark of Parkinson's disease.

In addition, it is known that the disease process of Parkinson's disease begins long before motor symptoms are clinically visible. Many patients report to their doctors that they already experienced non-motor symptoms associated with PD, such as fatigue, constipation, and olfactory changes, several years before onset of overt symptoms.

Risk Factors for Parkinson's Disease

Researchers have been unable to identify specific causes of Parkinson's disease, but there are many theories regarding factors which may individually or in combination play a role in its development. These include:

- Age - Age is the most important risk factor for PD. As the population ages, the worldwide incidence of PD is expected to rise significantly.
- Genetic predisposition - Researchers have found gene mutations related to juvenile and Young-Onset PD. Recently, a new mutation was identified on the LRRK2 gene that is believed to be related to idiopathic PD (from an unknown cause). Other genes that have been identified include SNCA, PARKIN, and PINK1.

- Family history - According to the National Institute of Neurologic Disorders and Stroke (NINDS), approximately 15-20% of individuals with Parkinson's disease have a close relative who exhibited a parkinsonian symptom. Estimates are that family members of an individual with PD have three to four times the risk of developing PD than the general population. It is thought that if the right factors come together in an individual with a predisposition based on family history, that individual will develop Parkinson's disease.

- Oxidative damage - Free radicals (unstable molecules) circulating in the brain may cause oxidation, resulting in damage to dopamine-producing neurons. Some researchers refer to free radicals as endogenous toxins (toxins produced by the body).

- Toxins - Exposure to environmental toxins such as pesticides may cause degeneration of the dopamine-producing cells. It is known that exposure to the herbicide Paraquat™ elevates the risk for Parkinson's. Although not clearly understood, it appears that smoking lowers the risk of developing PD.

- Occupational exposure - There is a higher prevalence of PD among welders, farmers, cabinet makers, and clothes cleaners than among other occupations. Industrial exposure to heavy metals (such as iron, zinc, copper, mercury, and magnesium) and drinking well water with high levels of heavy metals, also elevate the risk of PD.

- Accelerated aging of neural cells - This theory proposes that for unknown reasons, the normal age-related death of brain cells is accelerated in patients with Parkinson's disease, causing the dopamine-producing cells to "age" and die faster than normal.

Diagnosis of Parkinson's Disease

Signs and Symptoms of Parkinson's Disease

Early identification of Parkinson's disease (PD) is often missed because the symptoms can be subtle and the progression of disease is typically slow. Individuals may complain of generally not feeling well, or feeling a little down, or being just a little shaky. Usually, it is friends or family who first notice that something may be wrong and who encourage an examination by a doctor.

There are four primary symptoms of Parkinson's disease, and they are known as *TRAP*:

- Tremor (shaking)
- Rigidity (muscle stiffness)
- Akinesia and Bradykinesia (impaired movement)
- Postural and Gait Instability (impaired balance)

Tremor

One of the earliest symptoms that individuals with Parkinson's display, is a tremor in a limb on one side of the body (*unilateral*), which is more noticeable at rest. The most common limb to be affected is the hand, and the tremor consists of a "pill-rolling" movement of the thumb and index or third fingers. Tremors can also occur in the tongue, lower jaw, or legs. Some PD patients report a feeling of internal shaking which is not visible to others. A resting tremor is present in 70-80% of people diagnosed with Parkinson's disease, and disappears with purposeful activity of the limb. Tremors are also frequently noticeable when individuals with PD are walking. Head tremor is not typically experienced as an early symptom of PD.

Tremor is often the primary symptom which spurs individuals to seek medical help, since it is so noticeable and can interfere with daily activities. Severity varies, but tremors almost always worsen with fatigue, stress, anxiety, excitement, apprehension, and cold weather. Tremors usually disappear during sleep. In older adults, tremors are less common. Approximately 25% of individuals with PD do not develop tremors.

Rigidity

Rigidity consists of increased tone or stiffness of the muscles and can occur in any limb, the neck, or facial musculature. Most patients with early Parkinson's disease do not report a feeling of rigidity, but rather may report feelings of vague aching or discomfort in a limb. However, when the physician manipulates the limb during the physical examination, signs of rigidity become evident. There is resistance to passive movement, which may be seen at any point while testing full range of motion of the affected limb. If a tremor exists in the rigid limb, one may see smooth movement replaced with a broken up, ratchet-type of action ("cogwheel rigidity").

When rigidity occurs in the face, it can cause the classic "mask-like" appearance associated with Parkinson's disease. Some patients report pain due to the rigidity of arms and shoulders. Rigidity is not a part of the normal aging process, so if an individual presents to a doctor with rigidity and improves with anti-parkinsonian drugs, it is most likely caused by Parkinson's disease. Rigidity is not as common a symptom as tremor in patients with Parkinson's disease.

Akinesia and Bradykinesia

Akinesia refers to a significant *reduction or absence* of spontaneous movement and *bradykinesia* refers to *slowness* of movement. Bradykinesia is more common than akinesia, and affects fine and gross motor function. It is experienced as a delay of movement initiation (e.g., taking the first step in walking) and slow response once the action begins (e.g., walking very slowly). It occurs frequently in PD and is usually reported to be the most distressing and troubling symptom, as it makes the simplest of tasks very time consuming. Bradykinesia interferes with many daily activities such as walking, dressing, household chores, and getting up from or sitting down in a chair. An especially frustrating aspect of bradykinesia is that it is unpredictable and can occur in the middle of an activity.

Bradykinesia is differentiated from non-PD related types of slow movement, where all movement is slow. Bradykinesia associated with PD is observable, for example, when individuals perform a repetitive fine motor function motion rapidly, such as opening and closing their hands. They may begin at normal speed, but the movements become progressively slower as muscle fatigue sets in. Bradykinesia can also be observed with other fine motor activities, such as eye blinking, or when writing, where letters become progressively smaller. Bradykinesia occurs in up to 75% of individuals with PD, and is usually *asymmetric*, occurring on only one side.

Bradykinesia is also experienced as difficulty with activities that require manual dexterity, such as fastening buttons; or in tasks requiring repetitive hand motions such as brushing teeth. In the face, bradykinesia is experienced as a decrease in facial expressions and/or diminished eye blinking. Some individuals with PD experience slowness in the muscles involved in swallowing, leading to a buildup of saliva, which could cause choking.

Postural and Gait Instability

Postural instability is a general term that involves gait changes and a stooped posture which affects balance. It is one of the *axial* (spine-related) symptoms of PD and involves the head and trunk, rather than the limbs. As a result of changes in posture and stability, turning or moving abruptly may cause individuals with PD to lose their balance and fall. Some individuals with PD lean forward or backward, also causing them to fall easily, especially if they are bumped. For some individuals, especially older adults, postural instability may be a later presenting symptom of Parkinson's disease. Gait changes include asymmetric slowness, shuffling, and reduced arm swinging.

Various studies of PD patients have shown that:

- Nearly 70% of patients with PD fall at least once a year.
- The average time from onset of PD until the first fall is approximately nine years.
- The greatest predictor of falling is having fallen in the previous year, not disease severity.
- In a group of PD patients without dementia that was followed to track the development and progression of postural instability and gait disturbance, 53% of the patients showed signs of postural instability at the beginning of the study, increasing to 88% at an eight-year follow-up.

To read more about postural instability and gait disturbances in PD, please click on the following link: http://www.ncbi.nlm.nih.gov/pubmed/18787879

Non-Motor Symptoms of Parkinson's Disease

While in the past, Parkinson's disease was considered to be primarily a motor disorder, clinical evidence clearly shows that there is a strong non-motor component to the disease. Non-motor symptoms of PD contribute significantly to reduced quality of life for PD patients and are the subject of extensive study. Estimates are that up to 80% of people with Parkinson's disease (PD) experience non-motor symptoms, most of which increase in intensity with progression of the disease. These complications become more and more disruptive in the tasks of daily life and significantly impact quality of life.

Non-motor features of PD appear to precede the appearance of motor symptoms by up to several years. Indeed, many patients report experiencing non-motor symptoms such as fatigue, depression, constipation, and olfactory changes many years before they are diagnosed with PD.

Non-motor symptoms of Parkinson's disease are categorized as including cognitive/psychiatric changes, autonomic (neurological) dysfunction, sensory dysfunction, sleep disorders, pain, and fatigue.

Cognitive/Psychiatric Dysfunction

Cognitive Impairment

Cognitive impairment is highly variable and may start early in the disease process for some patients with PD, while others may not notice any change until years have elapsed. Functions affected by cognitive impairment include:

- Executive function (the ability to organize cognitive processes, such as planning ahead, prioritizing, or shifting from one activity to another)
- Working memory (temporary storage and processing of information required for complex cognitive tasks, such as language learning, comprehension, or reasoning)
- Attention (the capacity to focus while excluding other stimuli)
- Visual-spatial dysfunction (orientation in space and movement)

Studies show that when diagnosed with PD, up to 35% of patients may have signs of cognitive impairment and up to 57% may experience cognitive impairment three years after diagnosis. Cognitive impairment is progressive in severity and the range of deficits becomes wider as injury to cortical tissue spreads. One study reported that 17 years after diagnosis, only 15% of surviving subjects was not cognitively impaired. Cognitive impairment is frequently related to the development of dementia, psychosis, depression, apathy, and fatigue.

Depression

Depression in Parkinson's disease is relatively common and may occur months or years before motor-related symptoms are apparent. Up to 20% of patients with PD report having had depressive symptoms even many years before Parkinson's was diagnosed. The risk of depressed people later developing PD is said to be two to three times higher than non-depressed people. Various studies have placed the incidence of depression among PD patients at between 12-90%, depending on patient inclusion and the criteria for diagnosis of depression. Depression may also be related to chronic pain, which affects many people with PD.

Symptoms of depression in Parkinson's disease include:

- Depressed mood
- Fatigue
- Reduced energy levels
- Reduced appetite
- Sleep disturbances
- Memory disturbances

The diagnosis of depression can be elusive since symptoms of classic depression (not related to Parkinson's disease) may overlap with symptoms of Parkinson's disease (e.g., mask-face, fatigue, low energy levels). Many symptoms of depression also overlap with symptoms of hypothyroidism (e.g., akinesia, mask-face, mood variations) which affects some Parkinson's disease patients. Depression can also appear as a side effect of some Parkinson's disease medications. It is generally believed that in most PD patients, the severity of depression is mild to moderate, but in patients with dementia, the severity of depression is notably greater. Suicide is typically not associated with depression in PD.

There is increasing evidence that depression is part of the disease process of Parkinson's disease, rather than exclusively a reaction to the stress of illness. The reduced dopamine levels found in Parkinson's disease patients have been shown to affect the balance of several other neurotransmitters in the brain, including *serotonin*, which plays a role in depression.

Depression is one of the most prominent non-motor features of Parkinson's disease and is associated with faster progression of motor symptoms, more rapid decline in cognitive function, poorer compliance with taking Parkinson's medications, and more difficulties in performing routine activities of daily living. Physicians usually probe further into the possibility of depression if patients complain of fatigue and reduced energy levels.

Anxiety

Anxiety is common among patients with PD, estimated to occur in up to 40% of cases. The underlying cause of anxiety is not clear and may be related to several factors, including stress of the illness, neurochemical changes of PD, anti-Parkinson's disease medication, and other, as yet unidentified factors.

A study of the association between anxiety and Parkinson's disease patients showed that:

- One-quarter of the survey group of PD patients were diagnosed with anxiety disorder
- Prevalent forms of anxiety were panic disorder, generalized anxiety disorder, and social phobia
- Depression was observed in 14% of patients with anxiety
- Severity of PD was positively associated with anxiety, but not the duration from onset of PD
- Patients with gait instability and postural dysfunction were more likely to experience anxiety than patients whose dominant symptoms were tremor-related
- Dyskinesia (movement impairment) and drug-related on-off motor fluctuation periods increased the risk of developing anxiety
- Patients with Young-Onset PD were more likely to experience anxiety than those with later onset of PD
- Anxiety lowered quality of life in the majority of the study's patients

To read more about anxiety and Parkinson's disease, please click on the following link: http://www.ncbi.nlm.nih.gov/pubmed/20461800

Dementia

Dementia, a steady, progressive decline in memory and other cognitive functions, is considerably more severe than cognitive impairment and is estimated to occur in approximately 40% of individuals diagnosed with Parkinson's disease. It usually appears in later stages of PD. One study published in 2003 in *Archives of Neurology* (vol. 60:pp. 387-392) showed that 17 years after diagnosis, approximately 78% of the subjects in the study had dementia. The greatest risk factor for development of dementia in PD is advancing age, not the age of onset, and estimates are that by 90 years of age, 80-90% of PD patients have dementia. The severity of dementia increases as additional cortical structures become affected by the progression of PD. Other risk factors may include the presence of mild cognitive impairment, severity of PD, postural instability, gait disturbance, and speech problems. The risk of individuals with PD developing dementia is six times higher than that of the general population. It is estimated that 3-4% of people with dementia have PD.

Risk factors for Parkinson's disease-related dementia include:

- Advanced age (age 70 or older)
- A score of 25 or higher on the Parkinson's Disease Rating Scale
- Adverse psychological response to treatment of PD with levodopa
- Exposure to severe psychological stress
- History of cardiovascular disease

In an article published in *Neurology* in 2014 (Volume 83, pp.1253-1260), researchers reported the results of a prospective study the goal of which was to identify prominent nonmotor features of Parkinson's disease that may be predictive for dementia. This study, performed in Canada, included 80 patients with Parkinson's disease with an average disease duration of 10-years. At the start of the study (baseline), all 80 study subjects were dementia-free as evaluated by neuropsychological testing that measured executive function, attention, memory, and visuo-spatial performance domains using standardized tests. The subjects were then followed for a mean time interval of 4.4 years during which they were evaluated through a comprehensive assessment of physical and mental variables that focused on motor function, blood pressure, sleep disorders, and sensory function (odor and color discrimination).

Of the 80 subjects followed during the course of the study, 27 or 34% developed dementia. In general, those subjects who developed dementia were older and predominantly male. In addition, the following variables were also associated with a higher risk for dementia in Parkinson's disease:

- Cognitive impairment detected at the start of the study period
- Sleep disturbances detected at the start of the study period

- Decrease in orthostatic blood pressure during the course of the study
- Abnormal color discrimination during the course of the study

The researchers also noted that some motor function variables were also associated with the development of dementia in Parkinson's disease. These motor variables included:

- Gait abnormalities
- Falls
- Episodes of "freezing" while walking

In summary, this study found that specific motor and nonmotor features of Parkinson's disease can strongly predict the later development of dementia. Since this study included a relatively small cohort of only 80 subjects, additional studies involving a large number of Parkinson's disease patients are necessary in order to confirm the data from this smaller study. Identifying major predictive risk factors for dementia in Parkinson's disease would be a major advance since those patients who are deemed to be at high-risk for developing dementia may benefit from counseling, early treatment intervention, and planning for their future care.

A different medical condition known as *dementia with Lewy bodies* presents with dementia and parkinsonian features. It is distinguished from Parkinson's disease by the presence of other associated clinical features (cognitive fluctuations and visual hallucinations) and its progression over time. In dementia with Lewy bodies, the interval between the onset of parkinsonian symptoms and dementia is one to two years, while dementia associated with Parkinson's disease typically occurs ten years or more after the onset of Parkinson's disease.

Psychosis

Psychotic symptoms are one of the most common causes for hospitalization of PD patients and for placement in nursing home facilities. Psychotic symptoms include:

- Illusions - An illusion is a misinterpretation of what one experiences in the environment, such as seeing a rope as a snake.
- Delusions - Delusions are beliefs that are not consistent with reality (e.g., that a visiting relative is an imposter).
- Hallucinations - Hallucinations are perceptions of things that don't exist, such as seeing a car parked on an empty street, or smelling odors that are not there. Hallucinations can be simple or complex, and rarely occur before the initiation of dopaminergic drug treatment; they are therefore believed to be closely linked to medication. Risk factors for hallucinations may include:
    - duration of PD

- severity of PD
- advanced age
- cognitive impairment
- visual disorders

Autonomic Dysfunction

The autonomic nervous system controls involuntary body functions such as blood pressure, heart rate, temperature regulation (sweating), and gastrointestinal processes. Autonomic disturbances are increasingly recognized as PD-associated symptoms. Disturbances are associated with increased disease severity, higher doses of dopaminergic medication, and advanced age.

Examples of autonomic nervous system disturbances in patients with Parkinson's disease include:

- Constipation
- Frequent urination
- Drop of blood pressure
- Skin problems
- Dysphagia (difficulty in swallowing)
- Drooling
- Nausea and vomiting

Constipation is common among Parkinson's disease patients and is thought to occur in up to 60% of cases. It is due in large part to the general slowdown of gastrointestinal function and may also result from or be exacerbated by side-effects of PD medication. Patients experience different forms of constipation, which may include difficult, infrequent (fewer than three per week), or incomplete defecation. Stools may be lumpy or hard. Constipation has been reported to predate the onset of PD in some patients by as many as 20 years.

Frequent urination is caused by a sense of fullness in the bladder, resulting in individuals experiencing a frequent urge to empty the bladder during the day or night.

Drop in blood pressure tends to occur with positional change (e.g., sitting to standing) and is called *orthostatic hypotension*.

Skin may become excessively dry or oily especially on the face and scalp. There may be a reduction of sweating, or recurrent episodes of drenching sweats.

Dysphagia (difficulty swallowing) affects up to 85% of patients with advanced PD and leads to weight loss, a significant problem for patients with Parkinson's disease. Due to the difficulty swallowing, it takes individuals with PD a long time to complete meals and requires greater effort to eat and drink. An additional danger caused by dysphagia is the risk for choking, which reduces the incentive of some people for eating, causing further weight loss. Dysphagia and choking are also responsible for the high rate of aspiration pneumonia, caused by inhaling a foreign body (such as food, liquid, saliva) into the lungs. Aspiration pneumonia is the most common cause of death among PD patients. Dysphagia can occur during the "on" phase when it is related to dyskinesia, or during the "off" phase, when it is related to rigidity and diminished motor function.

Drooling is reported to occur in up to 75% of individuals with PD and is a source of significant embarrassment that leads to social isolation for many of the affected individuals. The actual production of saliva is typically normal, but due to motor impairment of the muscles involved with swallowing, the saliva pools in the mouth, resulting in drooling. In early PD, drooling occurs mainly while sleeping, due to muscle relaxation. As PD progresses, drooling intensifies. It is generally agreed that the severity of drooling corresponds to the severity of PD.

Nausea, vomiting, and other intestinal symptoms such as bloating, early satiety, and heartburn, occur more frequently in PD patients than in the general population and are related to PD itself, as well as to effects of many of the anti-Parkinson's medications, especially dopamine-related drugs. The gastrointestinal muscles are affected by PD, resulting in slower digestion and slower emptying of digested foods from the stomach to the small intestines and successive digestive organs, and this may be the source of many gastrointestinal symptoms.

Sexual Dysfunction

According to the National Parkinson's Foundation, approximately 81% of men and 43% of women report reduced sexual activity with increasing severity of Parkinson's disease. Many men report sexual dissatisfaction because of erectile dysfunction, thought to affect approximately 30 60% of male PD patients. Sexual dissatisfaction in women is related to the quality of their sexual experiences, poor body image, vaginal tightness, and urinary difficulties, such as an increased urge to urinate or urinary incontinence.

Sensory Dysfunction

- Loss or reduced sense of smell (hyposmia) - Olfactory deficits may start years before the diagnosis of PD and include problems with odor detection, odor differentiation, and odor identification. Odor dysfunction is persistent and is not affected by medication. Researchers are investigating the possibility that odor dysfunction may be due to a lesion in the olfactory tract in the brain. Individuals with idiopathic hyposmia (reduced smell due to an unknown cause) may be at a higher risk for PD later in life.

- Visual disturbances may appear in the absence of eye disease or poor visual acuity. Patients may have problems distinguishing objects that are the same color in anything less than very bright light. The reduction of visual contrast can interfere not only with daily activities but also in not seeing objects on the floor, causing patients to fall.

Sleep Disturbances

Sleep disturbances affect up to 70% of Parkinson's disease patients at varying stages of the disease and with varying intensity. There are several types of sleep-related problems, most of which arise either as a result of pathological changes in the brain, such as cell loss around arousal centers in the brain, responsible for sleep and wakefulness, or as side effects of medications used for treating PD.

Sleep disturbances include:

- Insomnia - Patients may have no trouble falling asleep but have difficulty staying asleep at night and/or cannot fall back asleep if they wake up during the night. They also tend to wake up very early in the morning experiencing tremors or feeling very stiff due to the "wearing-off" effect of dopamine-based medication. It is estimated that up to 60% of patients with PD experience insomnia nine years after disease onset. One study reported that insomnia was associated with female gender, disease duration, and depressive symptoms.

- Excessive daytime sleepiness (EDS) - This appears to be an independent problem and not a result of fatigue or nighttime insomnia. It is thought to occur in up to 15% of patients nine years after PD onset, but other estimates are that 40% of PD patients may be affected. It is very disruptive and has a strong negative impact on quality of life since it affects many daily activities such as driving, reading, or socializing. Patients may take frequent naps during the day, often leading to added difficulty sleeping at night. One study reported EDS to be associated with age, gender (male), use of dopamine-agonist medication, and disease severity.

- Rapid Eye Movement (REM) sleep disorder - Also called *parasomnia*, individuals physically act out the dreams that occur during the REM stage of sleep. This can manifest itself as vocalizations, kicking, trying to choke another person, trying to move as if running, or striking out, thereby potentially causing injury to a spouse or caregiver sitting or sleeping next to them. REM sleep disorder is thought to be due to a lack of the normal inhibition of motor movement during REM sleep. Parkinson's disease patients with this sleep disorder are at increased risk of developing dementia with Lewy bodies later in the course of PD. Up to one-third of PD patients are affected by REM sleep disorder. The incidence of REM sleep disorder is associated with male gender, lower disease severity, and higher doses of levodopa medication. It is thought by some clinicians that REM sleep disorder may be another condition that occurs in many people several years before they are diagnosed with PD, and that up to 60% of people who exhibit REM sleep disorder may later develop PD.

- Restless leg syndrome (RLS) - Individuals feel the need to move their legs continuously at night, to the point of strongly impacting their sleep quality. RLS affects approximately 8 10% of all people over the age of 65. Some studies have shown that RLS may be present in 20 50% of patients with PD, but estimates vary widely.

Pain

It is estimated that more than half of patients with PD experience pain or discomfort, and some of those patients report that pain is their most significant problem.

The Parkinson's Disease Foundation (PDF) reports that there are several sources of pain in PD including:

- Musculoskeletal pain - This includes pain related to rigidity, lack of movement, mechanical stresses on the muscles due to postural abnormalities, shoulder stiffness ("frozen shoulder"), and contractures due to immobility of a limb. Pain in the hip, back, or neck is common.

- Dystonia - Severe, prolonged body twisting and postures results in what many PD patients identify as the most severe pain they experience. The spasms may affect the limbs, trunk, neck, face, tongue, jaw, swallowing muscles, and vocal chords. In addition, it may cause the toes to curl painfully, the arm to pull behind the back, or force the head forward towards the chest. In some patients, dystonia may be related to the "wearing off" of medication, and may be most severe in the morning when they get up.

- Akathesia - Extreme restlessness is a severe form of discomfort felt by many patients with PD. They cannot stay still and it severely impacts their quality of life since it is literally disabling. Individuals experiencing akathesia may not be able to sit still, lie in bed, drive a car, or remain socially active. If akathesia occurs at night, they may lose sleep. The PDF estimates that akathisia is related to medication in approximately 50% of cases.

- Neuritic pain - This pain is associated with a specific nerve and occurs close to a nerve or nerve root. A common location is the L-5 lumbar root, which causes sciatica.

- Neuropathic pain - This pain results from generalized nerve involvement, rather than from one nerve (neuritic pain). Neuropathic pain is thought to be directly related to PD itself, and is described as abnormal sensations such as stabbing or burning pain that may occur anywhere in the body including the abdomen, chest, mouth, rectum, and genitalia.

Researchers in the United Kingdom published a study examining the prevalence and determinants of neuropathy in individuals with PD, and the roles of Vitamin B12 and levodopa exposure. There were 37 PD patients and 37 patients in the control group. Findings included:

- Neuropathy is more common in PD patients than in age- and gender- matched controls without PD (37% versus 8%).
- Vitamin B12 levels were significantly lower in patients with PD and neuropathy, than in individuals with neuropathy who did not have PD.
- In patients with PD and neuropathy, there was a significant correlation between cumulative levodopa exposure and vitamin B12 levels (longer exposure and lower B12 levels).
- Vitamin B12 deficiency was the most probable cause of neuropathy in patients with PD, and it may be related to exposure to levodopa.

The authors of this study suggest that perhaps vitamin B12 levels should be monitored in levodopa treated patients with PD. This study can be found at the following link: http://www.ncbi.nlm.nih.gov/pubmed/22049200

Fatigue

Fatigue in PD includes an overwhelming sense of tiredness and lack of energy that may occur in up to 75% of individuals diagnosed with PD. It appears to intensify as PD progresses, particularly in the presence of depression. Understandably, fatigue has a strong negative impact on quality of life, as well as on cognitive and physical functioning. Some patients report feeling strong fatigue many years before the motor symptoms of PD appear.

Some individuals may experience shortness of breath if the muscles of the chest cavity are affected by Parkinson's. Rigidity of the chest muscles may occur during "off" periods as the dose of medicine is waning, or during "on" periods when dyskinesia (involuntary movement) develops, resulting in insufficient expansion of the chest muscles.

In general, as PD progresses, the severity of motor and non-motor symptoms increases, as well. For example, falling becomes a greater problem as balance and walking deteriorate; or nighttime sleep disruption may increase due to frequent urination, muscular pain, and difficulty moving in bed, compounding the severity of fatigue. Each stage of PD requires careful evaluation in order to optimize quality of life for patients. In older people, quality of life may be even more affected because impairments that occur with the "normal" aging process compound the symptoms of Parkinson's disease. In advanced stages of PD, the need for allied supportive health professionals increases since more severe disabilities require more physical and emotional support.

A multicenter assessment of non-motor symptoms and their impact on quality of life in PD was published in 2009 in *Movement Disorders*. More than 1,000 patients were surveyed, and 98% of them had at least one non-motor symptom. The most common non-motor symptoms were:

- Psychiatric (68%) - anxiety was most common
- Fatigue (58%)
- Leg pain (38%)
- Insomnia (37%)
- Urinary symptoms (35%)
- Drooling (31%)
- Difficulty concentrating (31%)

The study authors noted that pain, fatigue, and psychiatric symptoms were significantly more common in women than in men, and that the prevalence of non-motor symptoms increased over the course of PD. A full-text copy of this article is available by clicking on the following link: http://www.ncbi.nlm.nih.gov/pubmed/19514014

Progression of Parkinson's Disease

As Parkinson's disease progresses, motor symptoms increase, strongly impacting quality of life. Studies report that up to 40% of patients with PD develop motor symptoms within four to six years following disease onset. Motor symptoms may appear as abnormal involuntary movements of the head, trunk, and limbs; motor fluctuations; or an overall decline in motor performance. The development of motor complications has been associated with younger age of onset of PD, increased disease severity, and higher doses of levodopa medication. Motor complications generally increase in severity and frequency with increasing duration of PD.

Many of the difficulties experienced by PD patients are related to the increasing severity of the four basic categories of PD symptoms: tremor, rigidity, akinesia, and postural instability (TRAP) including:

- Difficulty walking - Problems with walking can occur early or late in Parkinson's disease and include:
    - *festination* - This is an involuntary tendency to take small shuffling steps or "running steps" resulting in walking with increasing speed to prevent falling. It is often difficult for patients who are "running" to stop when they reach their destination. Festination is related to an abnormal center of gravity (due to postural changes) and is sometimes called a "catch-up" gait. It results from a combination of shortening of the stride while quickening the gait.
    - lack of arm swinging of one or both arms while walking - This contributes to difficulty walking, since the brain associates walking and arm swinging together so that when one is impaired, the other may be impaired as well.
    - stooped posture - This results from a greater contraction of chest muscles than back muscles. Exercise is very important to counteract tightening and muscle contraction, since stooped posture affects balance, can interfere with walking, and can result in falling and ensuing injury.
    - "freezing" - Freezing is a sudden, temporary inability to move one's legs or feet. It may present as a sudden inability to initiate or continue movement (e.g., walking). It frequently occurs when PD patients approach doorways while walking or turning, or when they are in an area with many people. Freezing is usually associated with visual cues, such as narrow doorways or spaces. It occurs during the "off" period when the effect of medication has worn off, and before the next dose of medication takes effect. It is a common side effect of dopaminergic medication. Freezing appears without warning and can last for several seconds. The duration and frequency of freezing episodes typically increase with the severity of PD. Freezing is one of the major causes of falling in patients with Parkinson's disease and occurs in approximately 30% of cases. Patients with early PD do not experience freezing as frequently as those in later stages of the disease. Risk factors for gait freezing include absence of tremor and longer disease duration. Freezing is strongly associated with other axial (spine-related) symptoms, such as postural instability. Anxiety can also play a role in initiating freezing or in preventing its resolution.
- Difficulties chewing and swallowing - Chewing and swallowing problems relate to

the overall symptoms of muscle rigidity and are caused by the:

- tongue - The tongue does not depress sufficiently to allow food to proceed to the throat.
- throat - Bits of food that are not completely swallowed collect in the throat and may fall into the airway, causing coughing or choking.
- esophagus - Muscles in the gastrointestinal tract, including the muscles involved with moving food down into the stomach from the esophagus, can be affected by PD, resulting in food chunks feeling like they are "stuck" or going down slowly. This can lead to heartburn or gastroesophageal reflux.

- Drooling - Excessive drooling occurs when saliva accumulates at the back of the mouth and, because of impaired musculature, is not swallowed. In addition to the embarrassment experienced by individuals who drool, drooling can also be dangerous since it can lead to aspiration of saliva into the lungs and cause choking or pneumonia.

- Loss of automatic movement (e.g., blinking) - This results in a limited range of facial expressions, or a "mask-like" appearance of the face.

- Speech impairment - Speech problems include a soft voice when speaking, slurring words, speaking too quickly, or hesitating before speaking. Speech impairment may be one of the first presenting symptoms of PD.

- Micrographia (progressively smaller handwriting) - This can appear at any stage of PD, but it often begins before other symptoms of Parkinson's disease are noticeable. The progression of symptoms in Young-Onset PD tends to be slower than for Adult-Onset PD. In addition, symptoms of Young-Onset PD, such as rigidity, bradykinesia, and dystonia (involuntary, often painful muscle spasms) usually begin symmetrically (on both sides) in the legs, whereas the first symptoms of Adult-Onset PD are usually asymmetrical (occurring only on one side).

Parkinson's Disease Rating Scale

Evaluation of motor severity and disability in Parkinson's disease (PD) is important as it is the only way available to chart the course of disease progression and to document the outcome of rehabilitation.

The progression of Parkinson's disease is usually documented using the Unified Parkinson's Disease Rating Scale (UPDRS), a rating scale introduced in 1987. There are three sections of the UPDRS which evaluate the major areas of disability in Parkinson's disease (cognition, behavior and mood; activities of daily living, and motor abilities), and one section of the UPDRS that evaluates complications of treatment.

- Cognition, behavior, mood (Part I)

    - intellectual impairment
    - thought disorder
    - motivation/initiative
    - depression

- Activities of daily living (Part II)

    - walking
    - speech
    - salivation
    - swallowing
    - handwriting
    - cutting food
    - dressing
    - hygiene
    - turning in bed
    - falling
    - freezing
    - walking
    - tremor
    - sensory complaints

- Motor abilities (Part III)

    - speech
    - facial expression
    - tremor at rest
    - action tremor
    - rigidity
    - finger taps
    - hand movements
    - hand pronation (rotation of the hands and forearms so that the palms face downward)
    - supination (rotation of the hands and forearms so that the palms face upward)
    - leg agility
    - rising from a chair

    - posture
    - gait
    - postural stability
    - body bradykinesia (slow movement)

- Complications of treatment (Part IV)

    - dyskinesia (difficulty in performing voluntary movements) - includes duration of dyskinesia, level of difficulty, and related pain
    - early morning dystonia (twisting and repetitive movements or abnormal postures)
    - "off-period" deterioration (period between two scheduled doses of levodopa medication when disease symptoms such as tremors, rigidity, and bradykinesia are more intense) - includes the *duration* of "off" periods, *predictability* based on dose, and the *pattern* of onset (sudden or gradual)
    - anorexia (including nausea and/or vomiting)
    - sleep disturbance
    - symptomatic orthostasis (difficulty remaining upright, typically due to a drop in blood pressure)

The UPDRS is administered by a health professional. Points are assigned to each area of disability or treatment complication based on patient response and physical examination. Parts I, II, and III contain 44 questions and each is measured on a 5-point scale; while part IV contains 11 questions and the scale ranges from 0 to 23. The cumulative score ranges from 0 (no disability) to 199 (total disability).

Diagnostic Testing for Parkinson's Disease

Currently, there are no blood tests or imaging scans to accurately diagnose Parkinson's disease (PD). The clinical diagnosis of PD is determined by evaluating symptoms and clinical presentation. It is very important that the examining physicians (usually neurologists) have the skill and experience needed to diagnose movement disorders, since Parkinson's disease is misdiagnosed in 25-35% of cases. The incidence of misdiagnosis declines sharply when individuals are evaluated by doctors who specialize in Parkinson's disease and other movement disorders.

The diagnosis of PD is difficult and, in some cases, may be a diagnosis based on the exclusion of other medical conditions. Typically, the neurological exam is the most revealing aspect of the overall diagnosis, but if exam results remain unclear, the physician may request laboratory or imaging studies in order to rule out diseases that present with symptoms that are similar to those of Parkinson's disease.

A diagnosis of PD is determined with:

- Patient history and physical examination
- Neurological evaluation
- Laboratory evaluation
- Imaging Studies

Patient History and Physical Examination

In addition to a physical examination, a detailed history of the onset of symptoms is a critical step in determining a diagnosis of PD. Relevant information includes:

- When symptoms first appeared
- Which symptom were first to appear
- History of non-motor symptoms
- Medication history
- Medical history
- Family history of Parkinson's disease or other neurodegenerative disorders
- Exposure to environmental toxins

Neurological Evaluation

Physicians perform in-depth neurological evaluations to determine which symptoms of TRAP (tremor at rest, rigidity, akinesia, and postural instability) are present, and their severity. However, these symptoms do not always present themselves in ways that clearly point to Parkinson's disease.

As described above, many physicians use the Unified Parkinson's Disease Rating Scale (UPDRS) initially to evaluate the presence and severity of symptoms, as it is a very sensitive indicator of signs of early Parkinson's disease, and of the presence Parkinson's disease symptoms in general. UPDRS evaluation results are derived from:

- Information collected from individuals and their family members regarding the *difficulty of performing routine activities* of daily living at home, such as bathing, showering, dressing, eating, and walking.

- Results of an intensive physical examination and neurological evaluation by the physician that focuses on the *presence and severity of TRAP symptoms* (e.g., getting out of a chair, walking with a normal stride, swinging the arms symmetrically).

Sometimes, to confirm a diagnosis of Parkinson's disease, the physician may prescribe an anti-Parkinson's levodopa-based medication to see if patients show improvement in walking, movements, or tremors. This information often rules out or establishes the diagnosis of Parkinson's disease, since most patients with classic PD respond to dopamine medication soon after it is initiated.

Laboratory Evaluation of Parkinson's Disease

Although there are no laboratory tests to establish definitively the diagnosis of Parkinson's disease, physicians may order any of the following tests in order to rule out other, underlying conditions:

- Complete blood count (CBC)
- Liver function test
- Thyroid function test
- Drug/Toxicology screen
- Serum and urine ceruloplasmin (for evidence of copper)
- Liver biopsy

Imaging Studies for Parkinson's Disease

If the diagnosis is still not clear after physical and neurological evaluation, physicians may order neuroimaging tests that reflect dopamine functioning, including:

- *Positron Emission Tomography* (PET Scan) in which a radioactive tracer such as 18-fluorodopa is injected intravenously while a scanner measures the uptake of the tracer in the substantia nigra portion of the midbrain and thus determines the number of dopamine cells present.

- *Single Photon Emission Computed Tomography with Dopamine Transporter* (DAT-SPECT) is similar to a PET scan but uses a different radioactive tracer and measures the uptake of the tracer in the brain differently than the PET scan.

PET and DAT-SPECT scans are rarely ordered since they are very expensive tests and are not always covered by medical insurance.

Differential Diagnosis of Parkinson's Disease

Several other conditions can mimic the symptoms of Parkinson's disease and must be excluded before the diagnosis is established. It is important to differentiate between true idiopathic (unknown cause) Parkinson's disease and parkinsonian symptoms that develop secondary to an underlying condition or medication.

The three most common categories of conditions that may be mistaken for Parkinson's disease include *medication-induced parkinsonism*, *Parkinson-plus syndrome*, and *essential tremor*.

- Medication-induced parkinsonism - Certain medications may either cause parkinsonian symptoms in non PD patients or may exacerbate the severity of symptoms in individuals diagnosed with Parkinson's disease. It is important to determine whether symptoms are related to medications, in which case discontinuing the medications can result in cessation of symptoms over time; or are indicative of actual Parkinson's disease. The most common medications that can induce parkinsonian symptoms include:

    - *antipsychotics* - Examples include haloperidol, thioridazine (Mellaril™), risperidone (Risperdal™), lithium (Eskalith™), chlorpromazine. (Thorazine™), and olanzapine (Zyprexa™). Parkinsonian side-effects of these medications can last one to two years after stopping the medications.
    - *antiemetics* - Drugs used to treat nausea and vomiting, such as prochlorperazine (Compazine™) and metoclopramide (Reglan™).
    - *antihypertensives* - Drugs used to treat high blood pressure, such as methyldopa (Aldomet™) and reserpine (Harmonyl™).
    - *antianginals* - Drugs used to treat angina or chest pain, such as dilitiazem (Cardizem™).
    - *antineoplastics* - Drugs used to treat various types of cancers.

- Parkinson-Plus syndromes - This is a group of disorders which presents with parkinsonism in association with other distinct clinical features, such as autonomic disturbances (Shy-Drager syndrome) or ataxia (Multi-System Atrophy). These syndromes show poor or short-lived therapeutic response to PD medications, and include symptoms or patterns of symptoms that do not appear in Parkinson's disease such as:

    - signs of dementia early after onset of symptoms
    - incidences of falling soon after onset of symptoms
    - feet set wide apart while walking
    - abnormal eye movements
    - symmetric (bilateral) signs of parkinsonism
    - severe disability within five years of onset of symptoms

- Essential tremor - tremors that are similar to those of PD but are identified based on the following characteristics:

- typically bilateral
- often accompanied by head tremor or tremulous voice
- handwriting that is typically large and tremulous
- signs of bradykinesia and rigidity are absent

Other conditions which should be ruled out when an individual presents with Parkinson's-like symptoms include:

- Multi-infarct disease (multiple small strokes), also called *arteriosclerotic* or *vascular parkinsonism*
- Other degenerative brain diseases - for example, Alzheimer's disease (destroys memory and cognition) and Huntington's disease (causes uncontrolled movements and cognitive loss)
- Dementia with Lewy bodies
- Normal Pressure Hydrocephalus - an excessive accumulation of cerebrospinal fluid in the cerebral ventricles of the brain
- Brain tumor
- Exposure to toxins such as manganese dust, carbon disulfide, and carbon monoxide
- Abuse of drugs containing MPTP (1-methyl-4-phenyl-1,2,3,6-tetrahydropyridine), often found in heroin, that causes a permanent form of Parkinson's. (This finding in the 1980's actually heralded an important breakthrough in Parkinson's disease research, as scientists could induce a simulated Parkinson's disease in animals for further study.)
- Shuffling gait disorders - may be caused by many other conditions and are often misdiagnosed as Parkinson's disease
- Wilson's disease - causes the body to retain copper

Clinical features of PD that distinguish it from these conditions include:

- Asymmetry of motor symptoms
- Tremors at rest
- Good to excellent response to levodopa-based medications

Treatment Options for Parkinson's Disease

Goals of Treatment for Parkinson's Disease

Treatment for Parkinson's disease is highly individualized. The goal of therapy is to reduce symptoms and improve quality of life while minimizing side effects of medications. The decision to treat early Parkinson's disease with pharmacological agents depends on the particular needs of patients and careful weighing of possible benefits, cost, and adverse outcomes. Doctors try to use the lowest dose of any medications to achieve satisfactory improvement of function.

At the present time, there is no universally accepted standard of care, either in terms of how to treat early symptoms, the optimum time to start treatment, or which medications should be given for initial treatment of Parkinson's disease. It is also difficult to set a standard of care because the response of each individual to medication can be so varied.

There is currently no cure for Parkinson's disease. With the initial diagnosis of Parkinson's disease, patients and their doctors must determine the level of discomfort or inconvenience of the symptoms in daily life and, based on these findings, establish the initial decisions for therapeutic intervention. There are four categories of treatment for Parkinson's disease, namely:

- Lifestyle modifications
- Pharmacological therapy
- Surgical therapy
- Experimental therapies

Lifestyle Modifications for Parkinson's Disease

There is general agreement that the first line of therapy for mild symptoms in early PD is lifestyle modifications. This approach alone, however, is usually not sufficient once the symptoms begin to interfere with activities of daily living. Lifestyle modifications effective for early PD include:

- Education
- Exercise
- Nutrition

Education

Individuals diagnosed with Parkinson's disease and their family members are encouraged to learn as much about PD as possible, including issues related to:

- Knowledge about the disease
- Signs of symptom progression and treatment options
- Variations in the rate of progression of disease
- Support services available in the community
- Emotional needs of individuals with PD and their caregivers
- Coping strategies for disabilities
- Help available for home care
- Respite care options

Exercise

Exercise is considered the most important adjunct therapy for all stages of PD. Exercise and physical activity are important in maintaining muscle strength, function and coordination. Physical therapists can teach new methods for standing, turning, and walking that maximize function and reduce the risk of falling. There are a variety of techniques for managing "freezing" that can significantly improve mobility and safety. Though exercise does not affect the progression of PD, it has a very positive effect on mobility and mood of patients. It also helps patients retain as much function and range of motion as possible in each stage of disease. Exercise should be carried out under the guidance of physical therapists who can respond to the changing needs of PD patients.

The types of exercises that are most important are:

- Aerobics
- Strengthening exercises
- Stretching exercises
- Balance training

Activities such as walking, swimming, or gardening are beneficial, and some researchers believe that weight-bearing exercises (such as walking) are especially helpful. Since energy levels fluctuate, it is important for individuals with PD to pace themselves when performing these activities. Balance training is crucial because postural instability increases with duration and severity of PD and raises the risk of falling and subsequent injury. There is also increasing evidence that exercise on a treadmill has a beneficial effect on gait as well as general well-being of individuals with Parkinson's disease. In addition, recent studies have highlighted the benefit of resistance training, weight-bearing exercise, and tai chi on improving motor symptoms such as gait and dyskinesia, as well as overall quality of life.

Exercise needs to be done consistently. Physical therapists suggest exercising for 20 minutes, three times a week, depending upon flexibility and fatigue level. Emphasis of exercise should be strengthening and stretching extensor muscles to counteract the flexors, which become rigid with disease progression. As Parkinson's symptoms progress, physical therapy plays an increasingly important role for maintaining limb mobility and range of movement.

In recent years, there has been growing interest in the use of exercise training to improve mobility and function in patients with Parkinson's disease, however, due to the inadequacy of data from rigorously controlled clinical trials, currently evidence-based guidelines for exercise in Parkinson's disease are lacking. In a study published in February 2013 in *JAMA Neurology* (Volume 70; Issue 2, pp. 183-190), researchers from the University of Maryland reported the results of a prospective, randomized clinical trial in which they evaluated and compared the efficacy of treadmill exercises and stretching and resistance exercises for improving gait speed, muscle strength, and fitness in 67 patients with Parkinson's disease. The patients were randomly assigned to one of the following 3 exercise groups: 1) high-intensity treadmill exercise - 30 minutes at 70% - 80% of heart reserve; 2) low-intensity treadmill exercise - 50 minutes at 40% - 50% of heart reserve; and 3) stretching and resistance exercises - 2 sets of 10 repetitions on each leg on 3 resistance machines (leg press, leg extension, and curl).

The major outcomes of this clinical trial were as follows:

- Improvements in gait speed as measured with a 6-minute walk test were observed with all 3 types of physical exercises. The largest improvements in gait speed, ranging from a 9% to a 12% increase, were noted with the lower-intensity treadmill and stretching and resistance exercises, respectively.
- Significant improvements in cardiovascular fitness (7% - 8% increase), as measured by peak oxygen consumption per unit time, were noted for both types of treadmill exercises but not with stretching and resistance.
- A significant increase in muscle strength (16%) was observed only for the patients in the stretching and resistance exercise arm of the study.

Although treadmill and stretching/resistance training were found to be beneficial for gait, fitness, and muscle strength, unfortunately, these benefits did not translate into improvements in daily function, activities of daily living, or quality of life. Nevertheless, the potential clinical effectiveness of combinations of treadmill and stretching/resistance exercises to alter or slow the course of disease progression in patients with Parkinson's disease should be explored in future rigorously controlled clinical trials.

Nutrition

It is important for individuals diagnosed with PD to eat a healthy diet with adequate fruits, vegetables, and whole grains to optimize health at every stage. In addition, vigilance regarding regular mealtimes and eating habits is necessary, since PD patients are at increased risk for weight loss and subsequent loss of muscle mass. Good dietary habits are also helpful in preventing or alleviating some gastrointestinal symptoms of PD, such as constipation.

Protein acts as a competitor with dopamine when it comes to being metabolized by the body. As a result, doctors recommend that PD patients not eat any protein for 30-45 minutes before and after taking levodopa-related medications.

Dietary supplements to treat the symptoms of PD have also been investigated. The position of the American Academy of Neurology is that there is no therapeutic or neuroprotective benefit to the nutritional supplement tocopherol (Vitamin E). However, there is ongoing investigation of the neuroprotective properties of Coenzyme Q10, a dietary supplement that is not regulated or approved by the U.S. Food and Drug Administration (FDA).

To read more about the position of the National Institute of Neurological Disorders and Stroke on Coenzyme Q10 and Parkinson's disease, please click on the following link: http://www.ninds.nih.gov/news*and*events/news*articles/pressrelease*parkinsons *coenzymeq10*101402.htm

Drug Therapy for Parkinson's Disease

Since the underlying disease process of Parkinson's disease involves the death of dopamine-producing cells and the subsequent reduction of available dopamine in the brain, one of the objectives of treatment is to increase the amount of available dopamine (also called *Dopamine Replacement Therapy*) by using agents that either:

- Increase dopamine levels in the brain
- Stimulate dopamine receptors in the brain
- Slow the metabolism and breakdown of dopamine in the brain, thereby reducing the fluctuations of dopamine in the blood

To meet these objectives, there are several categories of medication used for PD, namely:

- Dopaminergic agents (related to dopamine)
- MAO-B inhibitors
- COMT inhibitors
- Anticholinergics
- Cholinesterase inhibitors
- Antivirals

Dopaminergic Agents

Levodopa

Until recently, levodopa was considered the "golden drug" for initial symptomatic treatment of Parkinson's disease. Use of levodopa is also referred to as "dopamine replacement therapy". It became available in the 1960's and represented the first dramatic breakthrough in the treatment of Parkinson's disease. It is a highly effective drug and has been shown to extend life expectancy in Parkinson's disease patients. Before levodopa was introduced, the only agents that could relieve PD symptoms were anticholinergic drugs for the relief of rigidity and resting tremor. Levodopa is most effective for bradykinesia (slowness of movement) and rigidity. It is less effective for resting tremor. It is also not effective for posture, depression, and cognitive problems.

Levodopa brought about a revolution in Parkinson's disease treatment by reversing the neurochemical abnormality responsible for the symptoms and by making dopamine available for the brain. Dopamine itself cannot cross the blood/brain barrier (a tight "net" of blood vessels that protects the brain by barring entry of many chemicals into the brain). Levodopa was the first drug that was formulated in such a way that, when ingested orally, some dopamine was able to reach the brain.

Levodopa combined with carbidopa (Sinemet™) is the standard formulation of levodopa for Parkinson's disease patients today. This combination drug was a significant modification of levodopa because while carbidopa does not cross the blood brain barrier, it inhibits levodopa from being metabolized into dopamine in the digestive system (outside the central nervous system) and leaves a greater concentration of levodopa available to reach the brain with each dose. Thus, Sinemet™ reduces the amount of levodopa necessary to achieve desired motor control. Sinemet™ also minimizes some of the short-term side effects of pure levodopa, including nausea and vomiting. There is also a slow, controlled-release formulation of Sinemet™ that is available and that reduces side effects. However, it is only moderately effective and does not significantly reduce motor complications in most patients. Some doctors prescribe the controlled-release Sinemet™ to be taken as the last dose before PD patients go to bed at night.

Initial response to levodopa is usually quite dramatic. In fact, levodopa is considered to be so effective for Parkinson's disease that only approximately 10% of patients with Parkinson's disease do not respond. Indeed, some physicians are of the opinion that if a patient with parkinsonian symptoms does not respond to levodopa, other causes for the symptoms should be investigated.

Over time, patients taking increasingly large doses of levodopa find that not only is the effectiveness reduced, but major side effects become evident. This typically takes place in about 50% of the patients after approximately five years. Some of these events occur because levodopa has a short half-life (the time it takes for half the dose of the drug to be eliminated from the body) of approximately 1.5 hours, so the effect of the drug wears off quickly and symptoms reappear.

Side effects of long-term use of levodopa can have a profound effect on the quality of life of PD patients. They include:

- Dyskinesia - Involuntary movements (e.g., twitching, nodding, or jerking). The movements can be mild or severe, slow or rapid. The only way to control them is to cut back on the amount of levodopa being taken, but a return of Parkinson symptoms such as rigidity quickly recurs. At this point, other medications are utilized. This is the most problematic side effect of levodopa.

- "Wearing-off" effect - The deterioration of symptoms that occurs when levodopa wears off. It may be an indication that PD patients must take the drug more frequently. Often, patients experience symptoms of dystonia (involuntary muscle spasms which can cause abnormal movements) in the "wearing-off" period.

- "On-off" effect - Also called the "yo-yo" phenomenon, this is due to the fluctuation of dopamine levels in the blood. Patients experience sudden, unpredictable changes in the ability to move. They may go from carrying out a motor activity normally ("on") to suddenly freezing or becoming totally rigid with parkinsonian symptoms ("off"). This can happen several times a day. The "on-off" effect usually indicates either that the individual's response to levodopa is changing, or that the disease is progressing.

- Symptom intensity - Parkinsonian symptoms can be more intense before patients take the first dose of levodopa in the morning.

- Orthostatic hypotension - A drop in blood pressure when standing up after sitting.

- Hallucinations

- Restlessness

When levodopa is introduced to patients with Young-Onset Parkinson's disease, the response to the first dose is dramatic, but younger PD patients are likely to develop associated side effects, primarily dyskinesia, after a few months of taking the drug. Adult-Onset Parkinson's disease patients usually manifest the same long-term levadopa side effects after an average of three to five years.

Rytary

In January 2015, the U.S. Food and Drug Administration (FDA) approved RYTARY for the treatment of Parkinson's Disease. RYTARY is an extended-release oral capsule formulation containing both carbidopa and levodopa which is intended to reduce the amount of "off" time during the day when symptoms of Parkinson's disease are not adequately controlled. RYTARY consists of immediate-release and extended-release beads of carbidopa-levodopa in a ratio of 1:4 and, thereby, provides both immediate and extended blood levels of both drugs. The capsules may be swallowed whole or, for people who have difficulty with swallowing, the capsule may be opened and the beads sprinkled on applesauce and consumed immediately.

The FDA's approval of RYTARY was based on the results of two clinical studies involving a total of 774 patients with Parkinson's disease. The first trial (APEX-PD study) evaluated Rytary in 381 patients with early Parkinson's disease and found major improvements in both routine activities of daily living as well as motor function compared to placebo over a period of 6-months. The second trial (ADVANCE-PD) included 393 patients with advanced Parkinson's disease who were experiencing symptoms due to the wearing-off effect of their Parkinson medications. The results of this trial found that RYTARY significantly reduced the amount of "off" time and also increased the "on" time during waking hours by almost 2-hours compared to the immediate-release formulation of carbidopa-levodopa.

The following important safety information pertains to RYTARY:

- RYTARY should not be used in patients who are taking a monamine oxidase inhibitor medication, such as phenelzine or tranylcypromine, because of the increased risk of hypertension (high blood pressure) that may occur with the simultaneous use of both types of medications.

- RYTARY may cause some patients to become drowsy and sleepy when performing routine activities of daily living, including driving a motor vehicle.

- RYTARY should not be discontinued suddenly because sudden withdrawal of the drug may cause a constellation of symptoms that include fever, muscle rigidity, confusion, and problems with balance.

- The risk of cardiovascular ischemic events has been reported in patients taking RYTARY. Cardiovascular ischemia refers to problems with the circulation of blood to the heart muscle. A partial blockage of one or more of the coronary arteries can result in a lack of enough oxygenated blood (ischemia) thus causing symptoms such as angina (chest pain) and dyspnea (shortness of breath). A complete blockage of an artery causes necrosis (damage to the tissues) or a myocardial infarction, commonly known as a heart attack. Patients with a previous history of heart attack who have a residual irregular heartbeat (arrhythmia) should be monitored in a hospital during the period of initial treatment with RYTARY.

- RYTARY may increase the risk for hallucinations which may be accompanied by confusion, insomnia, and excessive dreaming.

- Psychosis may develop in patients treated with RYTARY. Psychosis may be associated with paranoid behavior, delusions, confusion, psychotic behavior, aggressiveness and agitation. For this reason, RYTARY in contraindicated in patients with a major psychotic disorder, such as schizophrenia.

- Patients taking RYTARY may be at increased risk for impulsive behavior and may experience intense urges such as the urge to gamble, spend money freely, or overindulge in eating. Reducing the dose of RYTARY may help to control these sudden and intense urges.

- RYTARY may also increase the risk of dyskinesia (involuntary muscle movements), upper gastrointestinal bleeding, and glaucoma.

Because RYTARY has only been available since early 2015, questions still remain about its optimal clinical use, particularly for neurologists who are considering switching a Parkinsonâ€™s disease patient from immediate-release carbidopa-levodopa (IR CD-LD) to RYTARY. In a recent article published in *Neurology* (Volume 86: Supplement 1, pp. S25-S35. 2016), two neurologists, Dr. Dee Silver and Dr. Richard Trosch, who combined have treated nearly 350 patients with RYTARY shared their experiences and provided guidance regarding important factors to take into consideration when contemplating a switch to RYTARY.

Here is a brief summary of their recommendations:

- RYTARY should be considered as an option for patients currently being treated with IR CD-LD who are experiencing bothersome levodopa end-of-dose wearing-off and dyskinesia symptoms.

- Although RYTARY is also approved by the FDA for the treatment of early Parkinsonâ€™s disease, most patients with early Parkinsonâ€™s respond well to IR CD-LD at 3 doses per day. However, RYTARY may be considered in patients with early Parkinsonâ€™s who are experiencing wearing-off symptoms despite a 3 to 4 times a day dosing schedule with IR CD-LD.

- When switching patients from IR CD-LD to RYTARY, it is important to inform them not stop taking their other Parkinsonâ€™s medications, such as a dopamine agonist, MAO-B inhibitor, or an anticholinergic medication, suddenly. The only change that should be made at this point due to documented wearing-off symptoms or dyskinesias is the switch from IR CD-LD to RYTARY.

- Dose adjustments are commonly needed for RYTARY which can usually be made within 3-weeks after starting the medication. The need to adjust the dosage will vary from patient to patient and depends on symptoms of â€œon-offâ€• fluctuations and dyskinesias.

- Switching to RYTARY requires patience on both the part of the patient and the physician. It may take 4 to 8-weeks for the benefit of the drug to be realized with a particular dosing regimen.

- The side effects or RYTARY are similar to those of IR CD-LD and include nausea, orthostatic hypotension, hallucinations, and delusions. Adjusting the dose of RYTARY can help reduce these adverse side effects.

Dopamine Agonists

Dopamine agonists mimic the effects of dopamine in the brain and cause neurons to react as if there were enough dopamine present to carry out their functions. This class of medications is used either as a monotherapy (single drug) or in combination with levodopa. If used initially as a single therapy, after a certain amount of time levodopa is added because the relief that the dopamine agonists provide is not sufficient to reduce the symptoms and improve the quality of life as the disease progresses. If levodopa is used as the initial therapy, the dopamine agonists are added in order to prolong the duration of time that dopamine is active in the brain and thus reduce the "wearing off" effect and resulting dyskinesia.

Dopamine agonists used to treat the symptoms of PD include:

- Ropinirole (Requip™) - used alone or with other medications
- Pramipexole (Mirapex™) - used alone or with other medications
- Bromocriptine (Parlodel™) - used alone or with other medications
- Apomorphine (Apokyn™) - used to treat "off" symptoms (such as difficulty moving, walking, and speaking) that occur as a dose wears off. Apomorphine does not prevent "off" episodes, but helps improve symptoms when an "off" episode has already begun.
- Pergolide (Permax™) - Withdrawn from the market in March 2007 by the U.S. Food and Drug Administration (FDA) because it has been linked to serious heart valve damage.
- Lisuride (Dopergin™) - not available in the U.S.

- Cabergoline (Cabaser™) - not available in the U.S.

Rotigotine (Neupro™ transdermal patch) is a dopamine agonist that is administered by applying a drug-treated patch to the skin once a day; the patch releases the drug through the skin over a 24-hour period. It was approved by the FDA in 2007 for use with early-onset PD, but was withdrawn from the market in the US in 2008 because of the formation of rotigotine crystals in the patches. When rotigotine crystallizes, less of the drug is available to be absorbed through the skin and, therefore, the efficacy of the product is variable. Neupro™ was reformulated and in June 2009, received approval for use for treatment of mild symptoms of PD in Europe. In April, 2012, Neupro™ was approved by the FDA, for the treatment of early and advanced Parkinson's disease.

While dopamine agonists are not as effective as levodopa, particularly in alleviating rigidity and bradykinesia, some doctors feel that since they do have some beneficial effects and their side effects are not as severe as those of levodopa, it is worthwhile to prescribe a dopamine agonist for mild symptoms initially, and then add levodopa later as needed. Some studies indicate that dopamine agonists as a monotherapy can reduce symptoms for up to three years and reduce the risk of developing side effects (dyskinesia and motor fluctuations) for up to four or five years. Another advantage of dopamine agonists is that they have a longer half-life than levodopa. Their use does not induce the "wearing off" effect or dyskinesia, and may actually moderate these effects when combined with levodopa.

Individuals with PD need to discuss with their doctors the advantages and disadvantages of taking levodopa or dopamine agonists.

In studies comparing quality of life in PD patients who took levodopa or dopamine agonists over a period of four years, the resulting quality of life scores were comparable, though there were fewer reports of dyskinesia for those patients taking the dopamine agonists (pramipexole or ropinirole). More long-term data is necessary before informed decisions can be made to reduce reliance on levodopa to treat the symptoms of Parkinson's.

Another major decision facing PD patients and their doctors is whether using dopamine agonists to delay dyskinesia and possibly delay disease progression is worth the poorer control of motor symptoms which are so effectively reduced by levodopa.

Finally, an important factor that doctors should consider before prescribing dopamine agonists is the burden of cost on patients, since dopamine agonists are significantly more expensive than levodopa.

Dopamine agonists do have some significant side effects, some of which are cognitive in nature and can significantly interfere with daily living. These include:

- Paranoia
- Hallucinations
- Confusion
- Nightmares
- Nausea
- Vomiting
- High risk-taking behavior, such as gambling
- Sexual obsession
- Sudden unanticipated sleep attacks

Some PD patients taking dopamine agonists develop dyskinesia as well, but these symptoms are usually not as severe as those seen following the use of levodopa.

Because of the nature of these complications, dopamine agonists are not given to patients who already suffer from any type of cognitive impairment. Recent data has shown a possible link between ergot-based dopamine agonists, such as bromocriptine (Parlodel™) and pergolide (Permax™), and dysfunction of cardiac valves. As a result, non-ergot based dopamine agonists such as ropinirole (Requip™) and pramipexole (Mirapex™) should be tried first.

In general, the data so far suggests that dopamine agonists are a significant addition to the arsenal of drugs that are effective in reducing symptoms of Parkinson's disease, as well as moderating the side effects associated with levodopa. However, because response to the drugs is so variable, doctors must evaluate carefully with their patients the choice of drugs, as well as the timetable for adding or combining new drugs.

Although some believe that there is a negative relationship between a high protein diet and dopamine agonists, data does not support that assumption.

Pramipexole On Underlying Disease (PROUD) Study

Pramipexole is a dopamine agonist medication that has been shown to be effective for improving motor symptoms in both early and advanced PD. Treatment with pramipexole in PD patients is started at the time that motor symptoms develop, up to now there have been no studies that evaluated the potential beneficial effects of pramipexole in people diagnosed with PD if given early in the course of the disease before motor symptoms become apparent clinically.

The Pramipexole On Underlying Disease (PROUD) study was the first clinical trial that was designed to evaluate whether early initiation of pramipexole therapy resulted in improved outcome in patients with PD. The study participants consisted of 535 adults diagnosed with early PD (within 2 years of the start of the study) who were randomly assigned to receive either pramipexole or placebo for a period of 15-months. Nine months into the study, the placebo group was switched to pramipexole. Improvements in outcome were evaluated with the unified Parkinson's disease rating scale (UPDRS) which measures behavior, cognition, mood, activities of daily living, and motor function. Neuroimaging studies were also performed on a subset of the study participants to measure striated dopamine binding in the brain as an indication of disease progression.

The results of the PROUD study showed that at 15-months, there were no statistically significant differences in the UPDRS scores between those patients given early pramipexole therapy and those given pramipexole on a delayed basis (placebo for 9 months then switched to pramipexole). Additionally, neuroimaging studies performed at 15-months showed an equivalent decrease in striatal dopamine binding between the early and delayed pramipexole groups. Based on the results of this clinical trial, the investigators concluded that on the basis of both clinical and neuroimaging measures, there is no evidence to support the hypothesis that pramipexole slows the progression of PD.

Tozadenant (SYN115)

Levodopa is a drug that is most frequently used to treat the symptoms of Parkinson's disease. Over the long term, however, many patients experience wearing-off motor fluctuations at least part of the day. The wearing off periods occur when the effects of a single dose of levodopa do not last as long as they used to. The wearing-off effect usually develops in patients who have been taking levodopa for several years. In an attempt to control the problem of motor fluctuations due to the wearing-off effect of levodopa, other medications such as MAO-B inhibitors and COMT inhibitors may be given along with levodopa. Since neither of these adjunct medications can completely eliminate the motor fluctuations resulting from the wearing-off of levodopa, there is a need to develop more effective medications that would reduce the wearing-off period.

Tozadenant (SYN115) is an oral medication that belongs to a class of drugs known as selective adenosine A2A receptor antagonists and has been shown to improve motor functions in animal models of Parkinson's disease. In a study published in 2014 in the journal *Lancet Neurology* (Volume 13; pp. 767-776) researchers reported the results of a randomized, double-blind Phase 2b multicenter clinical trial in which they evaluated tozadenant in levodopa-treated patients with Parkinson's disease who experienced at least 2.5 hours per day of "off-time" motor fluctuations. The clinical trial included over 400 Parkinson's disease patients who were randomized to receive either tozadenant in doses ranging from 60 mg to 240 mg twice daily for 12-weeks or a placebo. All of the patients had been taking levodopa for at least one year and were currently taking levodopa at least 4 times each day with a good response but were experiencing wearing-off motor fluctuations with at least 2.5 hours of "off-time" each day. To evaluate and compare the effectiveness of the treatments (tozadenant versus placebo), all of the study participants completed a Parkinson's disease diary prior to the beginning of the study and again at 2, 6, and 12-weeks (end-point of the study). The Parkinson's disease diaries were designed to measure the number of hours each day of motor fluctuations that each patient experienced due to the wearing-off effects of levodopa.

The major finding of this Phase 2b clinical trial was that oral tozadenant, at doses of 120 mg twice daily and 180 mg twice daily both significantly reduced levodopa off-time motor fluctuations by a little more than an hour each day compared to placebo. The most common adverse effects associated with oral tozadenant therapy in this trial were dyskinesia, nausea, and dizziness. The study authors concluded that tozadenant may be useful as an adjunct therapy to levodopa in patients with Parkinson's disease who experience off-time motor fluctuations. A Phase 3 clinical trial is currently in the planning stages to further evaluate the potential benefits of adjuvant tozadenant therapy in patients with Parkinson's disease.

Monoamine Oxidase Type-B (MAO-B) Inhibitors

There are two MAO-B inhibitors (MAOBIs) used in the treatment of Parkinson's disease, *selegiline* (Eldepryl™) and *rasagiline* (Azilect™). Dopamine is one of the brain chemicals known as *monoamines* which are broken down by a protein known as *oxidase*. MAOBIs limit the action of oxidase and prevent the breakdown of dopamine in the brain, resulting in an enhanced and prolonged effect of levodopa. There has also been considerable debate as to whether the MAOBIs used for Parkinson's disease are neuroprotective and possibly delay the progression of Parkinson's disease.

When taking MAOBIs, patients should be monitored on a regular basis for any changes in blood pressure. In addition, MAOBIs may interact negatively with some antidepressant medications so that PD patients being treated for depression should be carefully followed by a health care provider for any related complications. While taking MAOBIs, caution must be taken regarding adverse drug interactions with other medications, including many nonprescription cold medications that contain pseudoephedrine (a decongestant), and dextromethorphan (a cough suppressant).

Selegiline

The most widely used MAOBI is selegiline (Eldepryl™, Deprenyl™). Selegiline is used as an adjunct to levodopa since it increases the half-life of dopamine in the brain. There has been considerable debate as to whether selegiline is neuroprotective and possibly delays the progression of Parkinson's disease.

When given to patients in the early-stages of PD as a monotherapy, some studies suggest that selegiline delays the need for Sinemet™, possibly by as long as nine months. Other studies have shown that there is no support for giving selegiline as an initial monotherapy.

When given later in disease progression, selegiline boosts the effect of levodopa and improves the problem of fluctuations of motor response in about one-half to two-thirds of patients. The drug is easily tolerated. In general, selegiline is considered to be only moderately effective, resulting in its being prescribed more as an adjunct medication rather than as a monotherapy.

Side effects of selegiline include:

- Nausea
- Insomnia
- Confusion
- Abdominal pain
- Orthostatic hypotension (low blood pressure when changing from a sitting to standing position)
- Hallucinations (especially in the elderly)

Rasagiline

On May 17, 2006, the U.S. Food and Drug Administration (FDA) approved rasagiline (Azilect™) for use as an initial single drug therapy (monotherapy) for patients with early-stage Parkinson's disease, and in combination with levodopa in patients with moderate and advanced PD. Rasagiline is well tolerated and is not associated with side effects.

Azilect™ is a monoamine oxidase type-B (MAO-B) inhibitor drug that works by blocking the breakdown of dopamine. Azilect was approved in May 2006 by the U.S. Food and Drug Administration (FDA) for the treatment of Parkinson's disease. Azilect™ was originally approved by the FDA for use as a single drug (monotherapy) in patients with early Parkinson's disease and as an addition to levodopa in more advanced Parkinson's disease patients.

In June 2014, the FDA expanded the indication for Azilect™ to now include adjunct therapy with dopamine agonist medications. The new indication means that Azilect™ can be used to treat all stages of Parkinson's disease either alone or in combination with other Parkinson's medications. The FDA's approval for the expanded indication for Azilect™ was based on supporting clinical evidence from the ANDANTE study which showed that Azilect™ is also effective when used in conjunction with dopamine agonist medications.

Various studies have indicated that when used in levodopa-treated patients, rasagiline resulted in:

- Reduced motor fluctuations
- Reduced average daily "off" time

- Improved UPDRS scores for activities of daily living

Studies are ongoing regarding the possibility of rasagiline slowing the rate of progression of Parkinson's disease. While the results of several studies have shown benefits cited above, results regarding the neuroprotective aspect of rasagiline, i.e., that it slows the progression of PD, are not as clear, and have not yet been definitively supported by clinical trials. To read the results of a clinical trial in the *New England Journal of Medicine* of September 2009 that evaluated a delayed start of rasagiline in untreated PD patients, please click on the following link: http://www.ncbi.nlm.nih.gov/pubmed/19776408

A review of rasagiline and PD was published in 2012 in *Drugs*. The study author noted that two major studies in which rasagiline was given as a monotherapy, called ADAGIO and TEMPO, showed that rasagiline slowed the rate of worsening of symptoms as measured on the UPDRS. In addition, early initiation of rasagiline was associated with slower long-term progression than with later initiation. When rasagiline was given as an adjunctive treatment to levodopa in the LARGO and PRESTO studies, results showed that there was:

- Significantly reduced total daily "off" time
- Significant improvement of Clinical Global Impression (CGI) scores
- Significant improvement of UPDRS scores of activities of daily living during "off" time, and of motor scores during "on" time However, neuroprotective benefits were not clearly demonstrated. To read more about this review of rasagiline, please click on the following link: http://www.ncbi.nlm.nih.gov/pubmed/22439669

A study published in 2005 in the *British Journal of Cancer* (Volume 92, Issue 1; pp. 201-205) reported that Parkinson's disease patients may be at increased risk for developing a type of skin cancer known as *malignant melanoma*. This type of skin cancer was also diagnosed in a small number of patients treated with rasagiline. Although there is no clear evidence that rasagiline is associated with an increased risk of melanoma, current recommendations suggest that patients receiving treatment with rasagiline should be monitored for any signs of melanoma and other types of skin cancer.

Catechol-O-Methyltransferase (COMT) Inhibitors

- Tolcapone (Tasmar™)
- Entacapone (Comtan™)

COMT inhibitors (COMPTIs) prolong the effect of levodopa by blocking the enzyme known as catechol-O-methyltransferase (COMT) that breaks down dopamine in the liver and other organs. As a result, many of the adverse effects of levodopa which result because of sudden drops or fluctuations in the levels of levodopa, are reduced. This reduces the "off" duration which is seen in motor complications of levodopa. COMTIs also decrease the "wearing off" effect.

Tolcapone

Tolcapone (Tasmar™) is a potent drug which easily crosses the blood/brain barrier and which is used as an adjunct to levodopa. Because it increases the half-life of levodopa, patients can reduce levodopa intake by 25-30% when also taking tolcapone.

The major side effect of tolcapone is liver toxicity leading to liver failure. Because of this, tolcapone is given only to PD patients who are not responding to other medications. Once patients begin taking tolcapone, they require very close monitoring of liver function. The FDA suggests that patients be monitored every two weeks for the first year, then every four weeks for the following six months, and every eight weeks thereafter. The FDA also suggests that if patients do not exhibit substantial improvement within the first three weeks of taking the first dose, the use of this drug should be discontinued.

Other adverse effects of tolcapone may include:

- Dyskinesia
- Nausea
- Sleep disorder
- Muscle cramps

Entacapone

Entacapone (Comtan™) is similar in composition to tolcapone but does not cross the blood/brain barrier. It is also used as an adjunct to levodopa and is effective in reducing the "wearing-off" effect. Because of the lower risk of complications involved with this drug, it is the COMTI usually prescribed.

The main adverse effects associated with entacapone include:

- Urine discoloration
- Nausea
- Dyskinesia

Patients who have been taking levodopa often find that the Parkinson's symptoms recur and the dose required to achieve comfort may need to be raised. At that point, combining entacapone with levodopa and carbidopa in a drug called *Stalevo*™ has been found to prolong the action of levodopa, thereby providing symptom relief with lower doses of levodopa.

In a study published in 2009 in *Movement Disorders* (Vol.24(4):pp.541-50), 423 patients with early-stage PD were divided into two groups: one group received the combination medication Stalevo™ (levodopa/carbidopa/entacapone), and the other group received the combination drug Sinemet™ (levodopa/carbidopa). Results showed:

- Significantly greater improvement on the Unified Parkinson Disease Rating Scale (UPDRS) Part II for activities of daily living (ADLs) in the Stalevo™ group, compared to the Sinemet™ group.

- No significant differences on the UPDRS Part III (motor dysfunction) between the two groups.

- Wearing-off was observed in 29 subjects (13.9%) in the Stalevo™ group, versus 43 subjects (20%) in the Sinemet™ group.

- Dyskinesia was noted in 11 subjects (5.3%) in the Stalevo™ group, versus 16 subjects (7.4%) in the Sinemet™ group.

- Nausea and diarrhea were reported more frequently in the Stalevo™ group than in the Sinemet™ group. The study authors concluded that Stalevo™ provided more symptomatic benefit than Sinemet, without increasing motor complications.

On August 20, 2010, the FDA notified healthcare professionals that it is evaluating clinical trial data that suggest patients taking Stalevo™ may be at increased risk for cardiovascular events such as heart attack, stroke, and cardiovascular death, compared to patients taking Sinemet™. The FDA's decision to review the data of clinical trials was based on findings from the Stalevo Reduction in Dyskinesia - Parkinson's Disease or STRIDE-PD clinical trial, which reported a disproportionate number of heart attacks in patients treated with Stalevo™ compared to those receiving only Sinemet™. Although heart attack, cardiac irregularities, high blood pressure, and heart palpitations have also been reported with levodopa, previous clinical trials with Stalevo™ did not show an imbalance in heart attacks, stroke, and cardiovascular deaths.

At this time, the FDA's review of potential cardiovascular risks associated with Stalevo& #153 is still ongoing. In the meantime, until its review of the clinical trial data has been completed, the FDA has issued the following recommendations for healthcare professionals and patients:

- Healthcare professionals should regularly evaluate the cardiovascular status of patients who are taking Stalevo™, particularly if patients have a history of cardiovascular disease.
- Patients should not stop taking Stalevo™ unless told to by their healthcare professionals.
- The FDA will update the medical community and the public about its findings when

its review of Stalevo™ has been completed.

Comparison of Dopamine Agonists, MAOBIs, and COMPTIs

In July 2010, a review of the safety and efficacy of adjuvant drugs (add-ons) to levodopa for PD patients with motor complications was published in the *Cochrane Database of Systematic Reviews*. The review included results of 44 published trials involving 8,436 patients. The review authors compared dopamine agonists, COMTIs and MAOBIs to a placebo and to each other when added to levodopa.

When compared to a placebo, adjuvant therapy as a whole resulted in:

- Significantly reduced "off" time (up to 1.05 hours)
- Significantly reduced doses of levodopa
- Improved UPDRS scores (activities of daily living and motor functions)
- Adverse side effects that included constipation, dizziness, dry mouth, hallucinations, hypotension, insomnia, nausea and vomiting, and somnolence Data from indirect comparison of each of the drug classes indicated:

- Dopamine agonists were more effective in reducing "off" time, levodopa dose, and UPDRS scores than COMTIs or MAOBIs

- More dyskinesia was seen with dopamine agonists and COMTIs than with MAOBIs
- Overall incidence of side effects was greater with dopamine agonists and COMTIs than with MAOBIs, but the differences were of borderline significance.

The review authors concluded that while adjuvant therapy is beneficial for the symptoms noted above, dyskinesia and other negative side effects should be taken into consideration when considering which adjuvant medication would be most appropriate in each individual case.

To read more about a comparison of adjuvant therapies, please click on the following link: http://www.ncbi.nlm.nih.gov/pubmed/20614454

Anticholinergic Agents

Anticholinergic agents do not act directly on dopamine as do the other drugs previously mentioned. Rather, they block the effect of acetylcholine, a neurotransmitter that counteracts the benefits of dopamine in the brain. They are most effective for the control of tremor. Even so, they are only moderately beneficial. Examples of anticholinergic medications that may be used to better control tremor in patients with Parkinson's disease include:

- Trihexyphenidyl (Artane™)

- Benztropine (Cogentin™)
- Biperiden (Akineton™)
- Diphenhydramine (Benadryl™)
- Procyclidine (Kemadrin™)

Anticholinergics were the drug of choice for Parkinson's disease before the discovery of levodopa. Since only about half the people who take anticholinergics respond positively to them, and even then only for a brief time, they are not used often. Also, since tremors associated with Parkinson's are often not as severely disabling as other Parkinson's symptoms for many PD patients, there is less need to use this medication to control tremors.

Adverse effects associated with anticholinergic medications include:

- Dry mouth
- Nausea
- Urine retention
- Constipation
- Memory loss
- Confusion
- Hallucinations

Because of the nature of known side effects, anticholinergics are rarely prescribed for people over 70 years of age, or for individuals already experiencing mental impairment. In some circumstances, doctors find that older people who cannot tolerate anticholinergics may tolerate antihistamines (e.g., Benadryl™) and antidepressants (e.g., Elavil™) that have similar effects on Parkinson's symptoms. In general, anticholinergic drugs are not widely used in treatment of PD because of their minimal efficacy and the side effects associated with them.

Cholinesterase Inhibitors

Cholinesterase inhibitors are a class of drugs that slows the breakdown of the neurotransmitter acetylcholine in the brain, thereby increasing both its levels and duration of action in the brain. Acetylcholine plays an important role in learning and memory, and low levels of acetylcholine in the brain are associated with dementia and Alzheimer's disease. Cholinesterase inhibitors are used in Parkinson's disease to treat cognitive impairment and dementia.

Examples of cholinesterase inhibitors that may be used to treat Parkinson's disease-related dementia include:

- Donepezil (Aricept™)

- Galantamine (Reminyl™)
- Rivastigmine (Exelon™) - available either as an oral formulation (capsules) or as a transdermal patch designed for administration through the skin

Adverse effects of cholinesterase inhibitors include:

- Anorexia
- Nausea
- Vomiting
- Diarrhea
- Insomnia

Antiviral Drugs

The most commonly used antiviral drug is *amantadine* (Symmetrel™) which reduces symptoms of Parkinson's disease by blocking the re-uptake of dopamine and thereby increases the availability of dopamine in the brain. After several months of use, the effectiveness of antiviral drugs wears off in approximately one-third to one-half of PD patients. Amantadine is considered as only moderately effective for treating levodopa-induced dyskinesia, resulting in its being prescribed more as an add-on medication for PD, rather than as a monotherapy.

Side effects of amantadine include significant cognitive impairment (e.g., hallucinations). For this reason, it is usually not given to older people, or to people who already experience cognitive deficits.

Other negative side effects include:

- Blurred vision
- Depression
- Edema (fluid collection and swelling)
- Confusion

Medication Choices for Treatment of Parkinson's Disease

Treatment of PD patients is highly individual and is based on many criteria, including:

- Level of disability
- Stage of disease
- Age of patient
- Presence of comorbid conditions (e.g., dementia, hypertension)

Evaluation of these parameters helps determine when to introduce drug therapy and which classes of drugs to employ. Though there are no standard guidelines that are applicable for all PD patients, there are certain principles that seem to be widely accepted. These include:

- If patients are below the age of 70, treatment usually begins with dopamine agonists because dopamine agonists reduce the incidence of motor complications that are associated with levodopa.

- If patients are above 70 years of age, they usually begin treatment with levodopa because:

    - older patients are less likely to be affected by motor complications from levodopa
    - levodopa is less likely to cause problems for people with coexisting medical conditions
    - levodopa is better tolerated than most other classes of medications for PD and causes fewer cognitive and behavioral side effects
    - levodopa is typically the initial treatment for patients who are cognitively impaired

Beyond these general principles, there is a great deal of variation in how patients are medicated.

Decisions to raise or lower medication doses and to change or combine medications are made following careful consideration. It is therefore crucial for patients to be under the care of physicians who have extensive knowledge and experience in the diagnosis and treatment of Parkinson's disease, as well as the management of PD progression.

As the disease and level of disability progress, there are several options to manage motor complications that arise. These include:

- Smaller and more frequent doses of levodopa
- Adding or increasing dopamine agonists to levodopa
- Adding MAO-B or COMT inhibitors in order to increase the half-life of levodopa
- Adding amantadine or selegiline to reduce dyskinesia
- For PD patients who have problems with complex medication schedules, there are three options for once-daily medications, including cabergoline (Cabaser™), rotigotine patch (Neupro™), or the slow-release formulation of ropinirole (Requip™, Modutab™).

The Movement Disorder Society published an evidence-based medicine review update of treatments for motor symptoms of Parkinson's disease, which can be viewed at http://www.ncbi.nlm.nih.gov/pubmed/22021173

Neuroprotective Therapy for Parkinson's Disease

The goal of neuroprotective therapy is to prevent or delay the progression of PD by protecting the neurons from damage caused by biochemical changes that result in the loss of dopamine. The rationale for seeking neuroprotective therapy is that typically at the time of diagnosis with PD, approximately 40% of the dopamine-producing cells are still functioning, and it is important to protect them from injury. There are many studies being conducted to evaluate various potentially neuroprotective agents, but to date, no neuroprotective agents have proven effective in clinical trials.

Drugs and nutritional supplements being investigated as neuroprotective agents include:

- Selegiline and rasagiline - MAO-B inhibitors
- Pramipexole and ropinirole - dopamine agonists
- Coenzyme Q10 (ubidecarenone) - an antioxidant

A Practice Parameter published by the American Academy of Neurology (AAN) in 2006 indicated that no treatment has been shown to be neuroprotective. To read more about the conclusions of the AAN regarding neuroprotective agents and Parkinson's disease, please click on the following link: http://www.ncbi.nlm.nih.gov/pubmed/16606908

Neuroleptic Malignant Syndrome

Neuroleptic Malignant Syndrome (NMS) is a rare complication of Parkinson's disease and is usually triggered by a reduction or discontinuation of anti-parkinsonian drugs, especially, but not exclusively, levodopa. Additional triggers for NMS are infection and dehydration. Symptoms include high fever, increased rigidity and exacerbation of other Parkinson's disease symptoms, disturbances of consciousness, disturbances of the autonomic system (including blood pressure), and elevated creatine kinase levels in the blood.

It is critical for NMS to be treated immediately, as it can lead to pneumonia or renal failure. Treatments usually include infusion of intravenous fluids, cooling to reduce fever, increasing or reintroducing anti-parkinsonian medication, as well as administration of other drugs such as bromocriptine (Parlodel™) and dantrolene (Dantrium™). There is ongoing research into the efficacy of other medications in treating NMS.

Management of Non-Motor Symptoms of Parkinson's Disease

Non-motor symptoms of Parkinson's disease may be effectively managed using various modalities in addition to medication. Some of the symptoms that may be managed this way include:

Depression

Treating depression can often help people with Parkinson's disease cope better with the condition and can also improve their quality of life. The two most commonly used classes of prescription medications used to manage depression in people with Parkinson's disease are *tricyclic antidepressants* (TCAs) and *selective serotonin re-uptake inhibitors* (SSRIs). Although TCAs and SSRIs are commonly prescribed by both neurologists and psychiatrists to manage depression in patients with PD, currently there is a lack of sufficient evidence from randomized clinical trials to recommend one class of medication over the other. Some doctors prefer SSRIs because they are tolerated easily and do not affect mood or memory. TCAs cause orthostatic hypotension (drop in blood pressure when in changing positions) in some patients and have more side effects (e.g., dry mouth, blurred vision, and cognitive impairment). They also can be dangerous for patients with certain cardiac conditions. Some studies suggest that the dopamine agonist *pramipexole* is also effective for treating depression in Parkinson's disease.

In an article published in the March 10, 2009 issue of *Neurology* (Volume 72; pp. 886-892), researchers from the Robert Wood Johnson Medical School in New Jersey reported the results of a randomized, controlled clinical trial comparing the effectiveness of a TCA (nortriptyline) to an SSRI (paroxetine CR) in patients with Parkinson's disease. The study included 52 patients with Parkinson's disease who suffered from depression and who were randomly assigned to receive either nortriptyline, paroxetine CR, or a placebo over an eight-week period. The primary outcome evaluated in this study was an improvement in depression from baseline (before treatment) as measured using the Hamilton Depression Rating Scale, and the percentage of subjects in each group who responded to the treatments.

The researchers reported the following major findings from their study:

- Compared to placebo, patients who received a TCA (nortriptyline) experienced a significant reduction in depression as measured with the Hamilton Depression Rating Scale.
- Compared to placebo, no significant reduction in the level of depression was observed for those patients who had received an SSRI (paroxetine CR).
- A head-to-head statistical comparison of the TCA (nortriptyline) versus the SSRI (paroxetine CR) showed that a significantly higher number of patients in the nortriptyline group (53%) experienced a 50% or greater reduction in their level of depression as compared to those treated with paroxetine CR.
- Test subjects receiving the TCA (nortriptyline) also reported significant

improvements in sleep, anxiety, and social functioning compared to those treated with paroxetine CR.

A recent clinical trial demonstrated the efficacy of a serotonin norepinephrine re-uptake inhibitor (SNRI) called *venlafaxine extended release*, and a selective serotonin re-uptake inhibitor (SSRI) called *paroxetine*, when compared to a placebo, for the management of PD-related depression. Neither agent worsened PD motor symptoms. The authors of the study suggested that these two agents should be considered as first-line treatments for PD-related depression. For more information, please click on the following link: http://www.ncbi.nlm.nih.gov/pubmed/22496199

Parkinson's patients who are diagnosed with depression may benefit from other several treatment options, including:

- Counseling in individual or group therapy sessions
- Consultation with social workers, psychologists, or psychiatrists who may be able to reduce depressive symptoms by helping patients identify sources of stress and anxiety and suggesting changes and readjustments in everyday life to reduce the sources of stress.
- Exercise (e.g., walking) or other physical activity, which not only impacts depression but has the added benefit of alleviating motor complications in some patients.

Although Parkinson's disease is primarily considered as a motor disorder that is characterized by symptoms such as tremors, slow movement, muscle rigidity, and impaired posture and balance, it is also recognized that it can also impact cognitive function and psychological well-being. In fact, it has been estimated that up to 50% of patients with Parkinson's disease have psychological disturbances, the most common of which are depression and anxiety. If not diagnosed and treated early, these mental disorders can significantly impact the quality of life of both the Parkinson's patient and their caregivers. Despite this fact, it has been estimated that only about 20% of people with Parkinson's disease who experience psychological disturbances actually receive treatment for their psychological illness.

In a study published in the journal *PLOS One* in 2013 (Volume 8; Issue 11, pp. e79510), researchers from Australia performed a meta-analysis of randomized placebo-controlled clinical trials in order to examine the effectiveness of current treatments for depression and anxiety in people with Parkinson's disease. A total of 9 clinical trials were selected for inclusion in this meta-analysis. The combined number of patients among these 9 studies was 450, of which 252 received treatment for depression and/or anxiety while 180 subjects received placebo and served as controls. The most commonly used classes of medications in these clinical trials were tricyclic antidepressants (TCAs) and selective serotonin reuptake inhibitors (SSRIs). Some of the patients included in these trials also received alterative treatments, including Omega-3 fatty-acid supplementation and cognitive behavioral therapy.

When the data from all 9 clinical trials was combined or "pooled" for the meta-analysis, there was no statistically significant benefit noted in favor of either TCAs or SSRIs over placebo in the treatment of depression or anxiety in patients with Parkinson's disease. Although not statistically significant, both types of medications resulted in moderate improvements in controlling symptoms of depression and anxiety compared to placebo. The study also found that, as a class, TCAs were more effective than SSRIs for the treatment of Parkinson's associated depression.

Of particular interest was the finding that treatment of depression with Omega-3 fatty-acid supplementation or cognitive behavioral therapy was associated with a statistically large improvement in symptoms of depression and anxiety compared to placebo. Omega-3 fatty-acid supplementation is currently not recognized as a standard treatment for depression or anxiety and much more research is needed to confirm it's effectiveness in the treatment of these disorders. Cognitive behavior therapy, on the other hand, is recognized as an effective treatment for depression and anxiety in the general population and may also represent an option for Parkinson's disease patients who either do not respond to or cannot tolerate treatment with antidepressants or SSRIs.

In summary, psychological disturbances such as depression and anxiety are common in people with Parkinson's disease, however, only a relatively small percentage of patients receive treatment for these psychological disorders. In most cases, the first-line treatment of choice is usually SSRIs because they are associated with less severe side-effects than TCAs. The use of TCA's is usually considered for those patients who do not respond to SSRIs. Cognitive behavioral therapy should be considered as a potentially effective alternative method for the treatment of depression and anxiety in patients with Parkinson's disease based on its effectiveness for the treatment of these disorders in the general population.

Drooling

While anticholingeric drugs, such as glycopyrrolate (Robinul™), are helpful for some people to manage drooling, they have several side effects including constipation, urine retention, and cognitive impairments, especially in older patients. Other effective management options include chewing gum, sublingual atropine drops, and medications with anticholingeric effects, such as amantadine (Symmetrel™). Although not approved by the FDA, botulinum toxin (Botox) is recommended for its positive effect on drooling in many patients. It is administered as an injection into each parotid (salivary) gland in the base of the mouth. Preliminary studies indicate that Botox injections decrease drooling for up to 30 weeks.

To reduce nighttime drooling, patients may be advised to sleep in a more upright position rather than lying down. PD patients can also be taught to swallow more frequently than before, especially while eating, and speech therapists can show PD patients how to strengthen the muscles used in swallowing. When the drooling becomes pronounced, some doctors prescribe levodopa or dopamine agonists if not already being used, though their benefit is limited.

Dysphagia

Dysphagia (difficulty swallowing) typically does not respond to dopaminergic treatment, leaving aspiration (breathing in food, drink or saliva) as a major risk for these patients. In order to minimize the risk of aspiration, patients should try eating while in the "on" phase of medication and in a sitting position with the head tilted slightly downward. Food texture is important. Individuals should eat foods that have a uniform texture, use fluid thickening agents for liquids, take small bites, and gently cough after swallowing each bite. Evaluation and treatment recommendations by a speech therapist are beneficial.

Speech

Speech therapists evaluate various parameters of speech that may be affected by PD (e.g., volume, voice quality, and hurried speech) and provide suggestions for optimizing and improving them, as well as methods to improve communication. Some patients may choose to undergo an experimental procedure where collagen is injected into the vocal folds of the larynx to enhance vocal quality.

Pain

Pain in PD is a significant problem and is treated by pinpointing, whenever possible, the source of the pain. Treatment may include introducing dopamine agonists, modifying the dose of medication that patients may already be taking, the use of painkillers or antidepressants, or deep brain stimulation.

Sleep Disturbances

Since sleep disturbances may be related to Parkinson's disease medications, physicians may adjust dosages or even change medications. If PD patients have problems with excessive daytime sleepiness, a stimulant such as Ritalin™ may be recommended.

Modifications in the sleeping environment that may reduce disturbances include:

- Use of satin sheets because they are smooth and may make it easier for PD patients with stiff muscles to move or get comfortable in bed

- Use of well-placed pillows to help PD patients stay in a comfortable position and prevent rolling back into an uncomfortable position

It is important for PD patients to discuss changes in sleep patterns with their health care providers, since lack of restful sleep can cause significant interference in daytime and nighttime quality of life, not only for PD patients but also for their caregivers. Caregivers need to get an adequate amount of sleep to remain strong and supportive. Rehabilitation professionals should be able to make suggestions to help caregivers improve their sleep conditions.

Constipation

Constipation is one of the most common nonmotor features of Parkinson's disease and is estimated to affect between 20% to 30% of Parkinson's patients. Constipation can precede the classic motor symptoms of Parkinson's disease such as bradykinesia, rigidity, tremors, and shuffling gait by as much as 20 years. In most people with Parkinson's disease, constipation is due to decreased bowel movement frequency which may be attributed to the unusually slow transit of the waste material through the large intestine ("slow colonic transit") and/or difficulty with defecation. In addition to discomfort, chronic constipation can lead to potentially serious complications including bowel obstruction and bowel perforation. It is, therefore, important to diagnose and treat constipation as soon as possible before serious complications develop.

The initial approach for the management of chronic constipation in patients with Parkinson's disease involves relatively simple lifestyle modifications such as increasing dietary fiber and fluid intake along with encouraging non-intense aerobic exercises. If these conservative measures fail to correct the problem, treatment with medications may be initiated.

A recent article published in 2015 in *Expert Opinion in Pharmacotherapy* (Volume 16; Issue 4, pp. 547-557) reviewed the management of constipation in patients with Parkinson's disease and provided the following guidelines:

Constipation due to Slow Colonic Transit

- Oral Laxatives

Oral laxatives are usually considered as first-line treatments for the management of constipation in the general population, including people with Parkinson's disease. Oral laxatives include:

- Bulk-forming agents such as psyllium or bran
- Osmotic agents such as polyethylene glycol, lactulose, or milk of magnesia.
- Stimulant laxatives such as bisacodyl, sodium picosulfate, or Senna leaves. Stimulant laxatives are usually reserved for patients who do not respond to either bulk-forming or osmotic stimulants. Stimulant laxatives are only recommended for short-term use because they may induce tolerance, electrolyte imbalance, and problems with gut absorption.

- Lubiprostone

- Lubiprostone is an intestinal chloride secretagogue medication that was approved by the U.S. Food and Drug Administration for the treatment of chronic idiopathic constipation in adults (2006) and for irritable bowel syndrome with constipation in women (2008).
- Lubiprostone is a fatty acid taken orally that facilitates the passage of softened stool through the gut. It has been shown to be effective for the relief of constipation, including patients with Parkinson's disease, and is usually well-tolerated by most individuals.
- The most common side effects reported with lubiprostone treatament included diarrhea, nausea, abdominal pain, flatulence, dizziness, and vomiting.

- Rectal Laxatives

- Rectal laxatives, also known as enemas, may be prescribed as a rescue measure for people with chronic constipation who fail to respond to oral laxatives.
- Rectal laxatives should only be used sparingly and only as the last resource for occasional acute episodes of severe constipation in people with chronic constipation.

Constipation due to Defacatory Dysfunction

The term *defecatory dysfunction* is used to describe people who have difficulty emptying their bowels completely. The causes of defecatory dysfunction, also known as outlet obstruction, vary but can develop is there is prolapse (bulging) of the rectum or muscle spasms. The treatment options for people with defecatory dysfunction, including those with Parkinson's disease, include:

- Injections of levodopa or apomorphine
- Biofeedback therapy
- Botulinum toxin type A injection into the puborectalis muscle

If you or a loved one with Parkinson's disease suffers with constipation, talk with your neurologist or primary care doctor about the treatment options. For many people, simple lifestyle changes or treatment with oral laxatives will help to relieve the problem and will also prevent more serious complications from developing.

Frequent Urination

Urologists evaluate this symptom and determine if frequent urination is due to medications, infection, comorbid symptoms of aging (e.g., enlarged prostate), or multi-system atrophy, a condition that shares many similar symptoms with PD such as slow movement, stiff muscles, and mild tremors. There are medications and modifications in daily life that can be suggested for addressing bladder issues as PD progresses.

A recent study evaluated the efficacy of botulinum toxin type A for the management of overactive bladder in patients with PD. The treatment was effective for all eight patients that were included in the study. More about this study can be seen at the following link: http://www.ncbi.nlm.nih.gov/pubmed/21791351.

Weight Loss

Parkinson's disease patients are particularly at high risk for weight loss and it is important to take steps to manage this issue before it affects their overall health. Weight loss is closely related to changes in musculature involved in swallowing that make eating more difficult and less pleasurable. As a result, patients eat less and do not receive adequate nutrition. Cognitive changes may also affect concentration, and patients may become very distracted during meals, creating difficulties for caregivers who are helping them eat.

Modifications can be made by speech therapists who may be able to help patients optimize muscle control for swallowing; by nutritionists who can teach patients and their families or caregivers to modify meal plans and optimize calorie intake to include fruits, vegetables, and whole grains; and by occupational therapists who can suggest ways to reduce patients' distraction during mealtime (e.g., using plain dishes without pattern or design).

Helpful suggestions may include:

- Supplementing meals with high calorie drinks
- Eating frequent, small meals
- Modifying the consistency of foods to minimize choking or coughing
- Reducing distracting factors in the environment during meals

Thirst normally diminishes with age, and PD medications can exacerbate the problem by reducing thirst, resulting in dehydration. Drinking adequate amounts of fluid is therefore a high priority for PD patients.

Shortness of Breath

Shortness of breath may be partially controlled by modifying dosage and scheduling of PD medications. Physical therapy is also important for optimizing tone and flexibility of the chest muscles.

Visual Disturbances

Modification of the environment may help minimize visual disturbances. Some suggestions include:

- Brighter lights
- Greater contrast of color between floor and furniture
- Greater contrast where there are changes on the floor (e.g., steps, rugs, etc.)

Vitamin D3 Deficiency

Vitamin D is a vitamin that helps the body to absorb calcium - a mineral that is essential for normal bone formation. Although the body produces vitamin D when the skin is exposed directly to sunlight, very few food substances naturally contain vitamin D. Among the best sources of natural vitamin D are fatty fish such as tuna, salmon, and mackerel. Because many people do not consume sufficient amounts of these naturally-rich vitamin-D containing fatty fish, vitamin D is added to other foods such as milk, cereals, orange juice, and yogurt. Vitamin D is also available as a dietary supplement in the form of either vitamin D2 (ergocalciferol) or vitamin D3 (cholecalciferol). Vitamin D is used to treat a variety of conditions such as vitamin D deficiency (rickets), weak or brittle bones (osteoporosis), and softening of the bones (osteomalacia).

In a study published in 2013 in *Neurology* (Volume 81; pp. 1531-1537), researchers from Harvard University reported the results of a study in which they measured the plasma levels of 25 hydroxy-vitamin D3, a marker of how much vitamin D is present in the body, in 388 patients with Parkinson's disease and 283 control subjects without Parkinson's disease. The researchers found that about 18% of the Parkinson's disease patients had vitamin D deficiency compared to only 9% of the control subjects. Most experts define vitamin D deficiency as a level of less than 20 ng/mL of 25 hydroxy-vitamin D3 in the plasma. A higher proportion of subjects with Parkinson's disease (47.2%) were also found to have insufficient levels of vitamin D (plasma levels of 25 hydroxy-vitamin D3 between 20 to 30 ng/mL) compared to 39.9% of the control subjects. Moreover, the researchers found a positive correlation between low plasma levels of 25 hydroxy-vitamin D3 and both the prevalence and severity of Parkinson's disease.

A major finding of this study was that about 18% of patients with Parkinson's disease have a deficiency of vitamin D - almost twice the rate of that found in control subjects of similar age without Parkinson's disease. It is well known that people with Parkinson's disease are at increased risk for fractures from falls that can have serious consequences in this generally elderly population. It is also well established that vitamin D plays a key role in maintaining bone health and reducing the risk of bone diseases such as osteoporosis and osteomalacia. Although this study did not examine the incidence of fractures in Parkinson's disease patients who were found to have vitamin D deficiency, previous studies have shown that vitamin D supplementation, at doses higher than 400 IU/day, can significantly reduce the risk of fractures in individuals ages 65 or older. At this point, it is not clear whether Parkinson's disease predisposes patients to vitamin D deficiency and no causative link has been established between these two conditions. This study does suggest, however, that people with Parkinson's disease are at higher risk for developing vitamin D deficiency and should be monitored and treated with vitamin D supplementation if vitamin D deficiency is found.

Surgical Therapy for Parkinson's Disease

Surgical intervention was relatively common for the treatment of Parkinson's disease before the introduction of levodopa. It then fell out of practice, but as new surgical techniques became available, surgery has once again become an effective intervention for subsets of Parkinson's patients.

Surgery may be recommended as a treatment for:

- Patients of any age with advanced-stage Parkinson's disease who are no longer responsive to medication and who suffer from disabling tremors or associated Parkinson's disease "off-period" symptoms, such as motor fluctuations or dyskinesia.

- Parkinson's disease patients of any age who have a significantly impaired quality of life due to PD-related motor symptoms.

- Young-Onset Parkinson's disease patients for whom drugs do not adequately control symptoms and who have no evidence of cognitive impairment or other medical problems.

Surgery is not curative and is intended only to relieve symptoms of Parkinson's disease. Since the symptoms that may warrant surgery are associated with advanced PD, surgical intervention has not been considered as an option for earlier stages up to now.

Currently, there are two types of surgical procedures that may be considered for Parkinson's disease patients:

- Ablation (destruction of tissue)
- Deep Brain Stimulation (DBS)

Both procedures target highly specific areas of the brain, but while ablation involves the destruction of the tissue, DBS provides electrical stimulation to the tissue without destruction. Ablation and stimulation are performed via needle-guided stereotactic brain surgery. Before surgery, patients undergo several imaging studies in order to pinpoint the target area and other structures that lie in close proximity. During the procedure, patients are not fully anesthetized since they need to respond to the surgeon's questions about the sensations they are feeling at particular moments. Their responses help the surgeon determine if the electrode is in the correct location, since incorrect placement results in "incorrect" sensations, such as seeing flashing lights. There is no pain involved in the actual placement of the electrode as there are no pain sensors in the brain itself. However, local anesthesia is given during the preparatory stages of accessing the brain.

There are three targeted areas of the brain in which these surgical procedures are performed:

- Globus pallidus internus (GPi)
- Subthalamic nucleus (STN)
- Thalamus

If surgery is recommended for Parkinson's disease, confirmation of coverage with health insurance carriers is important, since not all surgical procedures for PD are covered.

Ablation

This type of surgery involves the destruction of targeted brain tissue via delivery of radiofrequency energy. Until the 1990s, this was the most common type of surgery for PD, but it is no longer used as frequently, due to the high risk of complications and more effective surgical procedures that are available. There are two types of ablation surgery, *pallidotomy* and *thalamotomy*.

Pallidotomy

Pallidotomy is performed to treat:

- Peak-dose dyskinesia (uncontrolled movements that occur when levodopa is at its highest concentration in the blood)
- "Wearing-off" dystonia (muscle spasms at the lowest concentration of levodopa as the medication wears off)
- Bradykinesia and tremor

Pallidotomy involves the destruction of the part of the globus pallidus internus (GPi) that controls movement. A wire probe is inserted into the GPi under MRI guidance and the precise target location is identified. The probe is heated by radio waves to a temperature that destroys the tissue in the immediate area. Since the reduction and loss of dopamine cause overactivity in the GPi, destruction of part of the tissue restores the balance needed for controlled movement. Effects from the ablation are seen almost immediately.

Outcomes of pallidotomy are estimated to be 70-90% reduction of dyskinesia and 25-50% reduction of tremor, rigidity, bradykinesia, and gait disturbance. The dose of levodopa may be reduced following surgery.

Pallidotomy can be performed as a unilateral procedure where ablation is limited to the GPi on one side of the brain, or as a bilateral procedure. While bilateral pallidotomy is more effective for reducing dyskinesia, it is associated with a higher risk for complications involving cognition, speech, and swallowing; therefore, bilateral pallidotomy is rarely performed.

There are complications in approximately 10-20% of patients undergoing pallidotomy. Risks include the probe striking a blood vessel and causing a stroke, damaging adjacent areas, or causing weakness, visual deficit, and confusion.

Thalamotomy

Thalamotomy involves the ablation of part of the thalamus (a structure below the GPi). It is effective for PD patients for whom tremor is the only disabling symptom. The ablation can be unilateral or bilateral, but bilateral thalamotomy is associated with a higher risk of complications and is usually not performed. Thalamotomy is rarely recommended for patients with PD.

Complications include hemorrhage, stroke, worsening gait instability, speech problems, and risk of the probe damaging other major brain centers that are adjacent to the thalamus. However, patients who exhibit these gait or speech problems prior to surgery are still considered as candidates for thalamotomy.

Deep Brain Stimulation

Deep brain stimulation (DBS) is not a destructive procedure and does not ablate any tissue. Rather, an electrode is placed in the target location and is attached to a battery-operated programmable stimulator located in the chest wall, about the size of a stopwatch, that delivers continuous, high-frequency electrical stimulation to the brain. Deep brain stimulation is a procedure based on evidence that loss of dopamine leads to abnormal activity in the GPi and STN. When electrical stimulation is delivered to one of those areas (which are centers for movement control), the DBS effectively "paces" the cells, and blocks or overrides any abnormal electrical activity.

Deep brain stimulation treatment is most effective for levodopa-induced dyskinesias, tremor, rigidity, stiffness, slowed movement (bradykinesia) and walking problems. Candidates for DBS include patients in whom control of symptoms with medication is inadequate. Patients who previously underwent pallidotomy or thalamotomy are still considered eligible for DBS. Generally it has been noted that patients whose symptoms do not improve with levodopa are not responsive to DBS. Most PD patients will have to continue to take the medications they were taking for motor symptoms before the treatment, but the doses may be reduced.

It is estimated that 10-15% of PD patients are candidates for DBS. Ideal candidates include:

- People younger than 70 years of age
- Individuals who are otherwise healthy, both cognitively and medically
- People who are responsive to levodopa and other anti-Parkinson's medications
- People who experience dyskinesia, motor fluctuations, or medically refractory tremors

Consideration of which brain structure is targeted for DBS is partially based on the following factors:

- *GPi* - Stimulation of the GPi produces the greatest improvement for dyskinesia, and more moderate improvement for tremor, rigidity, bradykinesia, and gait disturbances. Some patients can reduce the dosage of levodopa following this surgery. This surgery is also effective for patients suffering from dystonia. Bilateral deep brain stimulation of the GPi is well tolerated by many patients. Overall results of GPi stimulation are similar to those following pallidotomy.

- *Thalamus* - Thalamic stimulation is most effective when the predominant symptom of PD is disabling tremor that is stronger on one side of the body. Thalamic stimulation is reported to significantly reduce tremor in approximately two-thirds of the patients undergoing the procedure. Bilateral stimulation is possible, but is associated with a higher risk of complications.

- *Subthalamic nucleus* - The STN has developed into a major target area for DBS and may, in fact, be the most effective location for alleviating symptoms of Parkinson's. Most motor features of Parkinson's disease, namely bradykinesia, tremor, and rigidity, improve with DBS of the STN. Some patients can reduce the dosage of levodopa following DBS. This procedure is performed primarily on patients with advanced and disabling Parkinson's disease, but ongoing studies are evaluating the efficacy for other PD patients as well. Advantages related to STN stimulation include:

- motor symptoms are estimated to improve 40-60% during "off" periods
- motor symptoms improve up to 10% during "on" periods
- levodopa dose may be reduced up to 30%, resulting in a reduction of dose-related dyskinesia
- bilateral stimulation is superior to unilateral stimulation, and is associated with only slightly increased risk of complications

Following surgery, patients are taught how to control the implanted stimulator in order to achieve maximum benefit of symptom control from the deep brain stimulator device. Patients can also turn the stimulator off. It may take several weeks of adjusting the stimulator and medication before the full effect of DBS is achieved.

A study was published in 2010 in the *New England Journal of Medicine* (Vol.362(22):pp.2077-91) that compared deep brain stimulation (DBS) of the GPi to that of the STN in 299 patients with Parkinson's disease. The primary outcome was change in motor function, and the secondary outcomes included self-reported function, quality of life, cognitive function, and adverse effects. Results indicated:

- Motor outcomes and quality of life scores did not differ significantly between the two groups

- DBS in the STN was followed by greater reduction in the amount of medication needed to control PD symptoms

- There was no difference in self-reported functioning between the two groups

- Levels of depression worsened after DBS of the STN, and improved after DBS of the GPi

- Slightly lower scores in speed of cognitive processing followed DBS of the STN

- Serious adverse effects occurred in 51% of patients following DBS of the GPi, versus 56% of patients following DBS of the STN. There were no significant differences between the groups at 24 months post procedures.

Deep brain stimulation versus "best medical therapy" was compared in a study that was published in 2009 in the *Journal of the American Medical Association*. Two hundred and fifty-five patients with advanced PD were divided into two groups, one of which received DBS while the other received best medical therapy for PD. Primary outcome was time spent in the "on" state without troubling dyskinesia, while other outcomes included motor function, quality of life, neurocognitive function, and adverse events. Six-month follow-up of the patients revealed that:

- 71% of patients undergoing DBS and 32% of patients undergoing medical therapy reported significant improvement of motor function.

- Significant improvement in "on" time without dyskinesia (an average 4.6 hours) was reported for the DBS group, versus no change for the medical therapy group.

- Significant improvement in overall quality of life scores was reported for the DBS group.

- Moderate to severe side effects for both groups included falls, gait disturbance, dyskinesia, motor dysfunction, balance disorder, depression, and dystonia. During the six-month follow-up, there were significantly more adverse effects for the DBS groups, particularly of fall, gait disturbance, depression, and dystonia. By the end of the six-month follow-up, most adverse events had resolved for both groups.

You can read more about this study at the following website:
http://www.ncbi.nlm.nih.gov/pubmed/19126811

The U.S. Food & Drug Administration (FDA) approved DBS of the thalamus for the treatment of tremor in 1997, DBS of the STN for Parkinson's disease in 2002, and DBS of the GPi in 2003. Before pursuing this treatment option, PD patients should clarify the coverage policies of their health insurance providers regarding treatment with DBS.

Possible complications of DBS include an electrode or wire leading to the battery becoming infected, or excessive bleeding that may occur if a blood vessel is penetrated. Stroke is also recognized as a risk factor of DBS. Hemorrhage or stroke occurs in approximately 1 3% of patients who undergo this surgical procedure.

The advantages of DBS in general include:

- Brain tissue is not destroyed
- Stimulation can be continuous or can be turned off and easily adjusted for changing situations
- Symptoms are controlled more effectively, due to more precise placement of the electrodes
- There is low risk of stroke or hemorrhage
- The risk of levodopa-associated dyskinesia is reduced

- Motor fluctuations between "off" and "on" states are "smoothed over" and not as pronounced

The WeMove organization (www.wemove.org) notes that as DBS is being performed more frequently, and rare but serious neuropsychiatric side effects are being observed (including the onset or worsening of depression and the depression-associated risk of suicide), a neuropsychological evaluation is recommended before performing DBS to identify patients with depression or those at increased risk for depression.

With the increasing duration (almost two decades) since the initiation of DBS as a treatment for the symptoms of Parkinson's disease, longer-term disease progression is being studied. A 20-year follow-up of DBS of the STN in 19 subjects with Young-Onset PD who were diagnosed with Parkinson's up to ten years before treatment, was published in 2011 in *Brain* (Vol.134(7):pp. 2074-2084). Results showed that clinical and neuropsychological performance progressively worsened over the course of follow-up:

- 86% of patients developed dysphagia
- 64% developed a history of falling
- 57% developed urinary incontinence
- 43% developed dementia
- Progressive worsening of motor symptoms was observed in the "on" period following medication and in the "on" period of brain stimulation
- Gradual decline of all cognitive domains was observed, including executive functions (e.g., planning, organizing, and strategizing), language, reasoning, and memory
- Significant efficacy for primary motor symptoms of PD was still reported following DBS and dopaminergic medication.

The study authors conclude that long-term data following DBS indicates that symptoms that are not responsive to levodopa become progressively worse and are a cause of significant disability for patients.

A 36-month follow-up study comparing the outcomes of DBS of the GPi and STN was conducted, with the primary outcome being motor function during stimulation. Secondary outcomes included quality of life and neurocognition. Result of this study concluded that:

- Motor function improved and was comparable for DBS of GPi and STN
- Health-related quality of life scores significantly improved at six months but those improvements dissipated over time
- Scores of Dementia Rating Scales declined faster for patients undergoing DBS of the STN than the GPi

The authors of this study concluded that the decline of quality of life and neurocognition scores reflected underlying disease progression. In addition, they suggest that these results indicate the importance of non-motor symptoms (e.g., cognition) in determining the quality of life of patients with PD. More information about this study can be viewed at: http://www.ncbi.nlm.nih.gov/pubmed/22722632.

An expert consensus and review of key issues relating to DBS for PD was published in 2011 in *Archives of Neurology* (Vol.68(2):pp.165-171). The conclusions of this expert panel were as follows:

- Good candidates for DBS include patients with disabling motor fluctuations and/or medically intractable tremor without significant cognitive or psychiatric problems.
- DBS should be performed at major medical centers by physicians who are highly experienced and skilled in this procedure.
- DBS is effective for levodopa-responsive symptoms, and those benefits are sustained for several years.
- STN and GPi appear to be equally effective for treating motor symptoms.
- A greater reduction of medication is associated with STN DBS than GPi DBS, but there also may be an association with worsening non-motor symptoms and falls.
- Ablative procedures (e.g. thalamotomy) should be reserved for a select group of patients.

More information about this expert panel's consensus statement can be seen at: http://www.ncbi.nlm.nih.gov/pubmed/20937936

Experimental Procedures for Parkinson's Disease

The numerous side-effects of dopamine-related medications, such as dyskinesia and "on-off" fluctuations, and the drawbacks of surgical intervention, have resulted in significant efforts to find other forms of management of PD that are more targeted and do not cause such distressing side-effects. One of the areas that shows promise is therapy at the cellular level. There are several experimental procedures relating to cellular therapy under active investigation for treatment of Parkinson's disease. They are not being used to "cure" PD; that is, they are not being used to reverse the cause of reduced dopamine production. These strategies aim primarily at replacing the missing dopaminergic cells that are responsible for PD symptoms.

Two of the experimental procedures now being investigated are:

- Fetal Cell Transplantation
- Gene Therapy

- Stem Cell Transplantation
- Retinal Cell Transplantation

Fetal cell transplantation is an experimental procedure in which fetal dopamine-producing brain cells are implanted in the brains of patients with PD. The goal is for the cells to begin producing dopamine in the recipient. The procedure is performed to restore dopamine levels in the brain and thus restore patients to a less advanced stage of Parkinson's disease. It was first performed in the 1980s, but ended when some patients undergoing the procedure developed disabling dyskinesia.

Several hundred fetal cell transplants have been performed with variable outcomes, ranging from no response to significant improvement in a select few recipients. Some recipients also experienced severe dyskinesia. The expected outcomes include better motor control during "on" and "off" periods, an increase of "on" time, and a reduction of rigidity and bradykinesia. Some patients were able to reduce the dose of levodopa following surgery. Trials show that the greatest benefit of fetal cell transplantation is for younger PD patients. Because of the risk of rejection of the foreign fetal cells, patients may be given immunosuppressive drugs indefinitely. Fetal cell transplantation is still considered experimental and the source of fetal cells is controversial for many doctors and patients.

Fetal cell transplantation is usually performed bilaterally, either in stages or simultaneously. Since not all fetal cells take effect when transplanted, an oversupply of fetal cells must be transplanted in hopes of reaching a critical mass of cells that will restore dopamine production. Benefits from the surgery are usually not seen for several months because the cells need time to propagate. Adverse effects include the risk of severe dyskinesia, and there is an approximately 1 3% risk of stroke or hemorrhage.

To read more about fetal cell transplantation and PD, please click on the following link:
http://www.ncbi.nlm.nih.gov/pubmed/20887880

Gene therapy involves the injection of genes (such as the glutamic acid decarboxylase or GAD gene) that control dopamine production into the neurons of the subthalamic nucleus. Results look promising and there are several clinical trials underway. Another type of gene therapy, *neurotrophic factor gene therapy*, may prevent or slow the degenerative process of PD, as well as strengthen the remaining dopaminergic-producing cells. Trophic (growth) therapy may even have the potential to alter the course of PD. Some of the neurotrophic factors being studied that are very promising include *glial cell-derived neurotrophic factor* (GNDF) and *neurturin* (NTN). Please click on the following links to read more about gene therapy and Parkinson's disease:
http://www.nlm.nih.gov/medlineplus/news/fullstory_90594.html and
http://www.ncbi.nlm.nih.gov/pubmed/21259269

Research of *stem cell transplantation* for PD is in the very early stages of development. Information about stem cell transplantation can be seen at: http://www.ncbi.nlm.nih.gov/pubmed/22457112

Another approach being investigated at some clinical centers is the *transplantation of retinal pigment cells* (found in the back of the eye) into the striatum of patients with PD. Retinal cells are dopamine-producing cells and thus have the potential to increase dopamine in the brain. Investigators have not yet been able to show any long-term benefit to this procedure.

Guidelines for the Treatment of Parkinson's Disease

Management of Parkinson's disease is complex and involves important decisions regarding not only the initiation of medications but also adjustments to treatments that address changes that occur as the disease progresses. Physicians and patients face issues such as which drugs to use first, monotherapy or polytherapy, when to combine drugs, timing for initiation of medication and adjustment of medication protocols, and consideration of surgical options. One rule that is universally accepted, however, is that medication is initiated at the lowest reasonable dose and then slowly increased (titrated) until symptom relief is achieved with tolerable side effects.

Initial Therapy for Parkinson's Disease

A Practice Parameter published by the American Academy of Neurology (AAN) in 2002, concludes the following regarding *initial treatment* for Parkinson's disease:

- First-line treatment of newly symptomatic Parkinson's disease patients should consist of either levodopa or dopamine agonists. Levodopa is more effective than dopamine agonists for symptomatic relief, but carries greater risks for dyskinesia.
- Sustained release levodopa provides no advantage over the immediate release form of the drug.
- Selegiline, while of limited symptomatic benefit, has no neuroprotective properties.

Therapy for Motor Fluctuations and Dyskinesia in Parkinson's Disease

The AAN published four additional Practice Parameters for the treatment of dyskinesia in Parkinson's disease in *Neurology* in 2006 (Vol.66(7): 983-995) in which the following conclusions were drawn:

- Highest level of recommendation for reducing off time is with entacapone and rasagiline. Second level recommendation is with pergolide, pramipexole, ropinirole, and tolcapone, and the third level of recommendation is with apomorphine, cabergoline, and selegiline.

- Present evidence cannot recommend the superiority of one medication over another for reducing "off" time. Sustained-release carbidopa/levodopa (Sinemet™) and bromocriptine are not effective in reducing "off" time.

- Amantadine (Symmetrel™) may be considered to reduce dyskinesia.

- Deep brain stimulation of the STN may be considered to improve motor function and reduce off time, dyskinesia, and medication usage.

- There is insufficient evidence to support or refute DBS in the globus pallidus internus (GPi) or thalamus for reducing "off" time, dyskinesia, or medication usage, or to improve motor function.

- Preoperative response to levodopa predicts better outcome for DBS of the STN

More information about the AAN Guidelines for treating dyskinesia and motor fluctuations can be obtained by clicking on the following link:
http://www.ncbi.nlm.nih.gov/pubmed/16606909

Therapies That Slow the Progression of PD or Affect Motor Function

- Levodopa does not accelerate disease progression.
- No treatment has been found to be neuroprotective.
- There is no evidence that any food additive or vitamin supplement improves motor function.
- Acupuncture may provide symptomatic benefit for motor and non-motor symptoms.
- Exercise may be helpful for improving motor function.
- Speech therapy may be helpful for improving speech volume.
- No manual therapy has been shown to be effective for improving motor symptoms.

AAN Guidelines for neuroprotective agents and alternative medicine therapies that slow motor function decline in PD can be obtained by clicking on the following link:
http://www.ncbi.nlm.nih.gov/pubmed/16606908

Management of Non-motor Symptoms

A Practice Parameter for management of non-motor symptoms of PD was published by the

AAN in 2010 and supported the following:

- Dementia - Clozapine (Clozaril™) (Level B) and quetiapine (Seroquel™) (Level C) can be used for treatment of psychosis but olanzapine (Zyprexa™) should not be used. Rivastigmine (Exelon™) can also be used for treatment of PD-related dementia. Rivastigmine is available either as an oral formulation (capsules) or as a patch designed for transdermal (via the skin) administration. Based on clinical experience, donepezil (Aricept™) and memantine (Namenda™) could also be considered.
- Depression - Tricyclic antidepressants (TCAs) or selective serotonin reuptake inhibitors (SSRIs) can be recommended.
- Drooling - Botulinum toxin can be recommended.
- Constipation - Polyethylene glycol (Miralax™)
- Erectile dysfunction - Sildenafil (Viagra™)
- Excessive daytime somnolence - Modanifil (Provigil™)
- Fatigue - Methylphenidate (Ritalin™)
- Periodic limb movement of sleep - Carbidopa/levodopa (Sinemet™)

More information about the AAN Guidelines for therapies for non-motor symptoms of PD can be obtained by clicking on the following link: http://www.ncbi.nlm.nih.gov/pubmed/20231670

Many protocols for the management of non-motor symptoms of Parkinson's disease are mentioned in the medical literature. One of the more recently published articles can be seen at: http://www.ncbi.nlm.nih.gov/pubmed/21872276

Prognosis for Parkinson's Disease

Parkinson's disease (PD) is a chronic, progressive condition that is associated with increasing disability of motor function, balance, mood, cognition, behavior, activities of daily living, and quality of life. With appropriate treatment, the average life expectancy of PD patients is considered to be the same as for people who do not suffer from Parkinson's disease; however, complications of advanced Parkinson's disease such as pneumonia, choking, or falling, can lead to earlier mortality. If left untreated, Parkinson's disease progresses to total disability and can be the cause of early death.

The progression of motor symptoms in Parkinson's disease is usually very slow, although this varies widely among PD patients. Over time, symptoms increase and their severity intensifies. Some symptoms are directly related to PD and some are related to side effects of medications used to treat PD. With proper treatment, patients can live productive lives for many years.

The major challenge for patients with Parkinson's disease is adapting to their progressive disability. With the initial diagnosis of Parkinson's disease, patients and doctors must determine the level of discomfort or inconvenience of the symptoms in daily life and, based on these findings, establish the initial decisions for therapy. There is no set "timetable" regarding treatment for Parkinson's disease, and important issues such as when to start medications, or when to add or change medications, are in part determined by assessment of the level of interference with daily life that the symptoms present. On the average, if initial symptoms are mild, up to three years may pass from the time of diagnosis to the commencement of therapy with levodopa or a dopamine agonist, and another three to five years may pass before side effects from the levodopa interfere with daily living.

Several classes of drugs are used to treat symptoms and there are several medications within each class of drugs that can be taken either alone (monotherapy) or together (polytherapy). Successful drug treatment is a delicate balance of correctly dosing medications to achieve relief of symptoms while keeping side effects at a tolerable level. When medication alone does not provide sufficient relief, there are surgical options available that not only provide relief for eligible patients, but in some cases also lead to lower doses of levodopa.

As symptoms of Parkinson's disease intensify, some PD patients may require caregiving beyond what family members can provide and the option of professional caregivers or different types of assisted-living arrangements may need to be investigated.

The American Academy of Neurology noted in its Practice Guidelines published in 2006 the following points regarding prognosis in Parkinson's disease:

- A rapid rate of motor decline is associated with:
    - older age at onset (57-78) and rigidity/hypokinesia as an early symptom
    - male gender
    - postural instability
    - gait disorder
    - comorbidities (such as stroke, visual impairment)
- Older age at onset and rigidity at diagnosis "probably" predict earlier cognitive decline and dementia.
- Tremor as an early presenting symptom predicts slow progression of PD, longer response to levodopa, and a relatively good prognosis.
- Dementia, older age at onset, and decreased response to dopamine medication may predict increased risk of placement in a nursing home as well as shorter survival.

The Role of Complementary and Alternative Medicine in Parkinson's Disease

There are increasing numbers of professionals who combine knowledge of conventional treatment of Parkinson's disease with knowledge of complementary and alternative medicine. Research in this field is very active. There are limited clinical trials regarding Parkinson's disease and complementary medicine; most information is based on anecdotal evidence. It is important that health care providers be notified if PD patients are using any alternative therapies, no matter how insignificant or benign they may seem.

To see the latest conclusions of the American Academy of Neurology regarding the use of alternative medicine for the treatment of Parkinson's disease, please click on the following link:

http://aan.com/professionals/practice/guidelines/Neuroprotective_PD.pdf

Some forms of complementary medicine that may be effective for management of Parkinson's disease include:

Antioxidants

As noted above, there are ongoing studies regarding *Co-enzyme Q10*, a vitamin-like antioxidant that may have protective benefits for persons with Parkinson's disease. To date, no supplement has been clinically proven to be effective.

Herbal Preparations

- Primrose oil for reducing tremors
- Passionflower for reducing agitation and insomnia
- Ginger for reducing nausea and vomiting from medications
- Milk thistle to enhance liver function by removing toxins from the body

Acupuncture

It has been established that acupuncture causes certain physiological responses in the body that many patients claim brings relief to various Parkinson's disease symptoms. A study was published suggesting the benefit of acupuncture early in Parkinson's disease and can be seen at http://www.ncbi.nlm.nih.gov/pubmed/20034437

Traditional Chinese Medicine

Traditional Chinese medicine therapy for Parkinson's disease focuses on establishing balance in the body through treatment of meridians (channels of energy), as well as by other modalities.

Massage Therapy

Many Parkinson's disease patients report muscle relief as well as other symptomatic relief with various types of therapeutic massage.

Yoga

Yoga promotes relaxation and muscle stretching, which some patients with Parkinson's disease find helpful.

Tai Chi

Tai chi is a martial art that uses slow, intentional, and controlled movements to relax and strengthen muscles. It has been shown in a recent study published in the *New England Journal of Medicine* to be more effective than either resistance training or stretching for balance and stability in patients with mild to moderate PD. Study subjects in the tai chi group and the resistance training group also experienced significantly fewer falls over the six month study period compared to individuals in the stretching group. More can be seen about the outcome of this study at http://www.ncbi.nlm.nih.gov/pubmed/22316445

Alexander Technique

The Alexander technique teaches people how to stand, hold themselves, and move differently in order to release unnecessary tension and acquire balance and mindful movement. It has been shown to be beneficial for PD patients and, in clinical trials, showed a sustained increase in the ability to carry out activities of daily living. A recently published review of the Alexander Technique and its benefit for PD patients can be seen at http://www.ncbi.nlm.nih.gov/pubmed/22171910

Bright Light Therapy

Bright light therapy involves the exposure of PD patients to high intensity white fluorescent lights once a day. It is based on the model that suppressing the release of melatonin, which is effective for the treatment of depression and sleep disturbances, may be also beneficial for individuals with Parkinson's disease. Small studies yielded promising results for improvement of tremors, UPDRS for I (behavior and mood), II (activities of daily living), and IV (severity of PD disability), and depression. More information about bright light therapy can be seen at: http://www.ncbi.nlm.nih.gov/pubmed/17516492

Quality of Life Issues and Lifestyle Interventions in Parkinson's Disease

As Parkinson's disease progresses, a multidisciplinary team approach is usually the best approach for maintaining the quality of life for patients. Team members may include family doctors, Parkinson's disease specialists, neurosurgeons, urologists, nurses, social workers, physical therapists, occupational therapists, speech therapists, nutritionists, and, perhaps even complementary medicine professionals, among others. Therapists have identified many changes and modifications that help individuals with PD adapt to each stage of their illness and prevent injuries, such as falling, so that they can continue to live as independently as possible and maintain a good quality of life.

Falling is a major risk for PD patients and it increases with disease duration and with age. Gait changes and postural instability leave individuals more vulnerable to losing their balance and falling.

Modifications within the home can be made in order to reduce or minimize the risk of falling including:

- Placing adequate lighting in each room with easy-to-reach light switches, and placing nightlights in bathrooms and along the route that PD patients use to walk from the beds to the bathroom. Bright lighting is especially important for areas around stairs and outside the home (front walk, backyard).
- Placing grab bars strategically around the areas where PD patients walk so that they can grab on if they feel insecure on their feet or if they are falling
- Bundling all electric cords and extension cords and securing them near a wall and out of the routes that PD patients may walk within the home
- Removing loose tiles or anything over which PD patients may trip and fall
- Marking bottom and top staircase steps with white, non-slip paint to make them easily identifiable
- Avoiding slippery floors. Linoleum, vinyl, and wood floors are easier for many PD patients to negotiate safely than waxed or polished stone floors.
- Avoiding carpeting or using a low-pile carpet so that PD patients' feet do not get caught
- Removing area rugs

General safety tips for the home include:

- Placing PD patients in bedrooms on the main floor to avoid using stairs
- Using bedrails to help PD patients get into and out of bed

- Using satin sheets or pajamas to make moving in bed easier
- Arranging furniture so that PD patients have plenty of space to turn around either when standing or when using a wheelchair
- Using modified chairs that make standing up and sitting down easier for PD patients
- Setting up kitchen workspace in a place where PD patients can sit down to work
- Using plastic bowls and measuring cups to minimize breakage if something falls during use
- Providing gadgets that are easy for PD patients to use, such as electric or battery-operated can openers, and specially modified utensils such as scissors, vegetable peelers, or knives
- Using a transfer bench or chair while showering
- Placing grip bars on the walls of the shower and next to the toilet

The diagnosis of Parkinson's disease has a significant impact on patients and their families. One of the best ways to cope with fear of the unknown is to take advantage of the several excellent resources available for education and support of newly diagnosed PD patients. Ongoing research has led to important developments in controlling symptoms and improving quality of life, and newly diagnosed PD patients as well as patients with longer duration of disease can all benefit from making themselves knowledgeable about what PD involves, its diagnosis, symptoms, treatment options, and where to turn for support.

Due to the progressive nature of PD, there are many points in time at which important decisions have to be made reflecting the progression and increasing severity of the disease - for example, when individuals with PD should stop driving. Progression of PD and side effects of medication eventually impact individuals to the point where it becomes unsafe to continue driving. The point at which patients should stop driving is a difficult decision. According to Parkinson's Resource (http://www.parkinsonsresource.org signs that driving skills may be diminishing include increased traffic tickets, tire damage from hitting the curb, small dents in the car from hitting posts while pulling into or out of parking spaces, getting lost frequently, and family members increasingly criticizing PD patients' driving.

Support groups are very helpful in providing venues for patients and their families to discuss their challenges and receive feedback and support from other patients who may have experienced similar difficulties. Members of support groups may also provide suggestions for coping with changes that patients encounter in home life, social circles, and professional settings. In addition, many patients feel more comfortable discussing issues in the security of a support group, rather than with their physicians. Support groups also help reduce the feeling of loneliness that many PD patients and their caregivers may feel.

Depression is a common complication of PD, and it is important to seek treatment for suspected depression as soon as possible. In addition to the treatments mentioned above for depression, it is also helpful for individuals with PD to stay socially active and involved with family and friends. A systematic review of determinants of health-related quality of life in Parkinson's disease was publish in 2011 in *Parkinsonism and Related Disorders* (Vol.17:pp.1-9). The authors concluded that depression was the most frequently noted determinant of impaired quality of life in people with PD. Disease severity and disability were also frequently identified as sources of reduced quality of life. Motor symptoms that were cited the most frequently as interfering with quality of life were gait impairment and those related to drug therapy (e.g., "on off" periods of medication effectiveness).

Dementia is about six times more common in elderly patients with PD than in the average older adult. Support groups can help PD patients and their families cope with the development of dementia by suggesting educational resources, as well as practical ways of managing difficult or unsafe behaviors that may develop.

The slow rate of progression on Parkinson's disease provides ample time for patients and their families or caregivers to focus on future planning while patients are still able to participate in the decision-making process. Long-term arrangements need to be made for issues such as:

- Arranging long-term health, life, and disability insurance policies
- Determining possible modifications to be made in the work environment to facilitate continuing employment
- Investigating plans for future care, such as a professional caregiver, assisted-living facility, or nursing home
- Contacting an attorney regarding estate planning and wills Elder care attorneys, social workers, and other medical and social service professionals should be able to assist in drawing up these plans.

New Developments

- Scientists are investigating ways to diagnose early signs of PD in people at elevated risk (e.g., first degree relative) even before symptoms appear. Neuroimaging studies of changes in various brain structures and function through use of PET and SPECT scans are very promising. Pre-Parkinson's changes that are also being investigated include reduced olfactory (smell) sensitivity, and rapid eye movement (REM) sleep behavior disorder. The *Parkinson's At Risk Study* now being conducted at the University of Pennsylvania is focusing on identifying strategies to evaluate individuals with olfactory changes for early-stage Parkinson's disease. For more information about this study, please click on the following link: http://www.parsinfosource.com.

- Investigation continues into the development of anti-Parkinson's drugs that will provide prolonged benefits, improve or prevent dyskinesia, and modify progression of the disease. For more information, please click on the following link: http://www.ncbi.nlm.nih.gov/pubmed/22035030 Some of the anti-Parkinson's drugs now being considered include:

    - adensodine 2a antagonists (istradefylline, preladenant)
    - levodopa/carbidopa intestinal gel
    - extended release form of levodopa/carbidopa
    - carbidopa subcutaneous patch
    - safinamide

- *Safinamide* is a new MAO-B inhibitor that has dopaminergic and non-dopaminergic mechanisms of action. Although results of studies so far have been inconsistent, clinical trials are in process to evaluate its efficacy in symptomatic relief for PD and potential neuroprotective effects. You can read more about safinamide at: http://www.ncbi.nlm.nih.gov/pubmed/21913224

- A clinical trial was conducted in Japan that investigated the efficacy of *istradefylline* in reducing "off-time" periods in PD patients with motor fluctuations. Three hundred and sixty-three patients were divided into three groups with one receiving 20 mg, one receiving 40 mg, and the third receiving a placebo. Results indicated a significant reduction of "off-time" in the groups receiving istradefylline (up to 1.5 hours) vs. placebo (.66 hours). The most common adverse effect was dyskinesia. To read more about this study, please click here: http://www.ncbi.nlm.nih.gov/pubmed/20629136

- Several clinical trials are underway investigating the efficacy of *melevodopa*, a derivative of L-dopa, in patients with advanced PD and motor fluctuations. Authors of a study published in Pavia, Italy reported significant benefit when melevodopa was used as an adjunct to Stalevo_™, namely, a significant reduction of total hours of "off" periods, especially in the morning and afternoon; and faster onset of "on" periods. You can read more about melevodopa by clicking on the following link: http://www.ncbi.nlm.nih.gov/pubmed/19935405

- *Zonisamide* is an anti-epileptic drug that has been the subject of three clinical trials in Japan that resulted in significantly improved major symptoms in patients with PD. Effects were maintained for more than one year even in patients with advanced PD. In animal models of PD, zonisamide was shown to have neuroprotective properties, but that has not yet been shown for humans. For more information, please click here: http://www.ncbi.nlm.nih.gov/pubmed/20629136

- Scientists are investigating alternative methods for delivering levodopa, thus avoiding many of the side effects that come with the fluctuation of levels of orally administered levodopa in the blood. Among the techniques being studied are implantable pumps that provide a continuous controlled supply of levodopa. Other models being investigated include medicated skin patches and implanting capsules of dopamine-producing cells into the brain. To read more about drug delivery systems that are used and that are under development, please click on the following link: http://www.ncbi.nlm.nih.gov/pubmed/19651197

- Additional non-oral drug delivery systems that are being investigated for the management of motor symptoms of PD can be seen at the following link: http://www.ncbi.nlm.nih.gov/pubmed/21314492 and include:

    - iontophoretic (delivery into the skin via pulses of electricity)
    - intranasal (medication injected into the nostrils)
    - inhaled (medication is inhaled into the nostril)
    - sublingual (medication is placed under the tongue)
    - direct delivery (surgical delivery of medication into the brain or cerebrospinal fluid, intraperitoneal delivery of medication directly into the gut, or microscopic implants)
    - intravenous delivery
    - enteral infusion (delivery directly into the gastric system)
    - subcutaneous (delivery of medication under the skin)
    - gene therapy (to be delivered directly into a specific location of the brain)

- Levodopa-carbidopa intestinal gel (LCIG) is undergoing continued investigation as an alternative to oral administration in patients with advanced PD. It is typically administered via percutaneous endoscopic gastrostomy (PEG). In a literature review published in 2011, researchers found that in patients who were infused continuously with LCIG, levodopa plasma levels were more stable than with oral levodopa. In addition, LCIG may significantly improve motor complications ("on-off" fluctuations and dyskinesia), motor scores on the UPDRS rating scale, non-motor complications, and health-related quality of life. While adverse effects are similar to those of oral levodopa, 70% of patients on LCIG experienced technical problems with the infusion device. The study authors suggest that LCIG may be considered as an alternative for DBS in patients for whom DBS is contraindicated. This study can be found at: http://www.ncbi.nlm.nih.gov/pubmed/21351823

- Investigators are studying the feasibility of genetically engineering cells (e.g., skin cells) that can be grown in the laboratory to produce dopamine, and then implanting them into the brains of patients with Parkinson's disease. A great advantage would be that cells would be readily available and also that the cells would be obtained directly from the Parkinson's disease patient, thereby eliminating the problem of immune system rejection. To read more about this exciting development, please click on the following link: http://journals.lww.com/neurotodayonline/Fulltext/2009/04160/PD_Patients__Skin_Cells_Reprogrammed_Into_Stem.1.aspx

- A new technique called *dorsal column stimulation* is being investigated as an alternative to deep brain stimulation (DBS) for the treatment of PD symptoms. The research is currently in early stages and is not yet being tested on humans, but appears to be promising. The National Institute of Neurological Disorders and Stroke (NINDS) published a description of *dorsal column stimulation* research at the following link: http://www.ninds.nih.gov/news*and*events/news*articles/news*dcs *parkinson*rats.htm

- Researchers reported that five late-stage Parkinson's disease patients showed significant improvement when the protein *GDNF* was introduced into the *putamen* area of the brain (which regulates movement) by a tube connected to a mini-pump. It reduced "off" time and reduced or eliminated dyskinesia. Some researchers see this exciting development as a potential vehicle to treat the underlying disease in addition to symptoms. This drug is still in very early stages of development and testing.

- Information regarding ongoing clinical studies can be obtained at the Clinical Trials Listing Service at http://www.centerwatch.com or at http://www.clincialtrials.gov

Questions to Ask Your Doctor about Parkinson's Disease

- What is my stage of Parkinson's and what treatments are appropriate at this stage?
- What follow-up is necessary?
- Do I have to restrict or change my daily routine?
- How will Parkinson's disease affect my employment?
- How should I prepare my employer for the changes that will have to be made to accommodate my disability?
- What diet and exercise regime should I follow?
- At what point should I begin taking medication?
- Which medication is most appropriate for my symptoms?
- What side effects should I anticipate from the medication(s)?
- At what point should I consider surgery?
- Will complementary medicine help my symptoms at the present stage?
- Who will assemble the team of allied health professionals that I will need and coordinate my care?
- What is the prognosis (outlook) for short and long-term?
- What resources are available to me and my family for education and support?
- Are there any clinical trials in which it would be appropriate for me to participate?

NOTES

Use this page for taking notes as you review your Guidebook

3 - Guide to the Medical Literature

Introduction

This section of your *MediFocus Guidebook* is a comprehensive bibliography of important recent medical literature published about the condition from authoritative, trustworthy medical journals. This is the same information that is used by physicians and researchers to keep up with the latest advances in clinical medicine and biomedical research. A broad spectrum of articles is included in each *MediFocus Guidebook* to provide information about standard treatments, treatment options, new developments, and advances in research.

To facilitate your review and analysis of this information, the articles in this *MediFocus Guidebook* are grouped in the following categories:

- Review Articles - 68 Articles
- General Interest Articles - 33 Articles
- Drug Therapy Articles - 12 Articles
- Clinical Trials Articles - 34 Articles
- Deep Brain Stimulation Articles - 13 Articles

The following information is provided for each of the articles referenced in this section of your *MediFocus Guidebook:*

- Title of the article
- Name of the authors
- Institution where the study was done
- Journal reference (Volume, page numbers, year of publication)
- Link to Abstract (brief summary of the actual article)

Linking to Abstracts: Most of the medical journal articles referenced in this section of your *MediFocus Guidebook* include an abstract (brief summary of the actual article) that can be accessed online via the National Library of Medicine's PubMed® database. You can easily access the individual article abstracts online by entering the individual URL address for a particular article into your web browser, or by going to the following special URL:

http://www.medifocus.com/links/NR013/0718

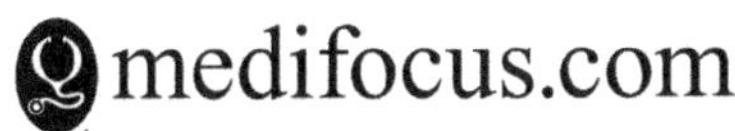

Recent Literature: What Your Doctor Reads

Database: PubMed <January 2015 to July 2018>

Review Articles

1.

The potential role of herbal products in the treatment of Parkinson's disease.

Authors: Amro MS; Teoh SL; Norzana AG; Srijit D
Institution: Department of Anatomy, Universiti Kebangsaan Malaysia Medical Centre, 56000 Kuala Lumpur, Malaysia. Lumpur, Malaysia. Lumpur, Malaysia. Lumpur, Malaysia.
Journal: Clin Ter. 2018 Jan-Feb;169(1):e23-e33.
Abstract Link: http://www.medifocus.com/abstracts.php?gid=NR013&ID=29446788

2.

The launch of opicapone for Parkinson's disease: negatives versus positives.

Authors: Castro Caldas A; Teodoro T; Ferreira JJ
Institution: a Neurology Service, Department of Neurosciences , Hospital de Santa Maria , Lisbon , Portugal. Portugal. University Hospitals NHS Foundation Trust , London , United Kingdom.
Journal: Expert Opin Drug Saf. 2018 Mar;17(3):331-337. doi: 10.1080/14740338.2018.1433659.
Abstract Link: http://www.medifocus.com/abstracts.php?gid=NR013&ID=29415596

Go to http://www.medifocus.com/links/NR013/0718 for direct online access to the above Abstract Links.

3.

Effects of physical exercise programs on cognitive function in Parkinson's disease patients: A systematic review of randomized controlled trials of the last 10 years.

Authors: da Silva FC; Iop RDR; de Oliveira LC; Boll AM; de Alvarenga JGS; Gutierres Filho PJB; de Melo LMAB; Xavier AJ; da Silva R
Institution: University of State of Santa Catarina, Center for Health Sciences and Sports, Adapted Physical Activity Laboratory, Florianopolis, Santa Catarina, Brazil.; University of Brasilia, Faculty of Physical Education, Brasilia, Brazil.; University of Southern Santa Catarina, Medicine Course, Florianopolis, Santa Catarina, Brazil.
Journal: PLoS One. 2018 Feb 27;13(2):e0193113. doi: 10.1371/journal.pone.0193113. eCollection 2018.
Abstract Link: http://www.medifocus.com/abstracts.php?gid=NR013&ID=29486000

4.

Pharmacological interventions for psychosis in Parkinson's disease patients.

Author: Friedman JH
Institution: a Movement Disorders Program , Butler Hospital , Providence , RI , USA. Providence , RI , USA.
Journal: Expert Opin Pharmacother. 2018 Apr;19(5):499-505. doi: 10.1080/14656566.2018.1445721. Epub 2018 Mar 1.
Abstract Link: http://www.medifocus.com/abstracts.php?gid=NR013&ID=29494265

Go to http://www.medifocus.com/links/NR013/0718 for direct online access to the above Abstract Links.

5.

Fatigue in Parkinson's disease: concepts and clinical approach.

Authors: Nassif DV; Pereira JS
Institution: Department of Neurology, Pedro Ernesto University Hospital, State University of Rio de Janeiro, Rio de Janeiro, Brazil. Rio de Janeiro, Rio de Janeiro, Brazil.
Journal: Psychogeriatrics. 2018 Mar;18(2):143-150. doi: 10.1111/psyg.12302. Epub 2018 Feb 6.
Abstract Link: http://www.medifocus.com/abstracts.php?gid=NR013&ID=29409156

6.

Towards stem cell based therapies for Parkinson's disease.

Author: Parmar M
Institution: Department of Experimental Medical Science, Wallenberg Neuroscience Center, Division of Neurobiology and Lund Stem Cell Center, Lund University, BMC A11, S-221 84 Lund, Sweden malin.parmar@med.lu.se.
Journal: Development. 2018 Jan 8;145(1). pii: 145/1/dev156117. doi: 10.1242/dev.156117.
Abstract Link: http://www.medifocus.com/abstracts.php?gid=NR013&ID=29311261

7.

Pimavanserin: novel pharmacotherapy for Parkinson's disease psychosis.

Authors: Sahli ZT; Tarazi FI
Institution: a Department of Psychiatry and Neuroscience Program , Harvard Medical School, McLean Hospital , Belmont , MA , USA. McLean Hospital , Belmont , MA , USA.
Journal: Expert Opin Drug Discov. 2018 Jan;13(1):103-110. doi: 10.1080/17460441.2018.1394838. Epub 2017 Oct 31.
Abstract Link: http://www.medifocus.com/abstracts.php?gid=NR013&ID=29047301

Go to http://www.medifocus.com/links/NR013/0718 for direct online access to the above Abstract Links.

8.

Pharmacokinetic drug evaluation of opicapone for the treatment of Parkinson's disease.

Authors: Svetel M; Tomic A; Kresojevic N; Kostic V
Institution: a Clinic of Neurology, Clinical Center of Serbia, Faculty of Medicine , University of Belgrade , Belgrade , Serbia.; b Clinic of Neurology , Clinical Center of Serbia , Belgrade , Serbia.
Journal: Expert Opin Drug Metab Toxicol. 2018 Mar;14(3):353-360. doi: 10.1080/17425255.2018.1430138. Epub 2018 Jan 24.
Abstract Link: http://www.medifocus.com/abstracts.php?gid=NR013&ID=29345156

9.

Spotlight on opicapone as an adjunct to levodopa in Parkinson's disease: design, development and potential place in therapy.

Authors: Annus A; Vecsei L
Institution: Department of Neurology, Faculty of Medicine, Albert Szent-Gyorgyi Clinical Center, University of Szeged. Center, University of Szeged; MTA-SZTE Neuroscience Research Group, Szeged, Hungary.
Journal: Drug Des Devel Ther. 2017 Jan 9;11:143-151. doi: 10.2147/DDDT.S104227. eCollection 2017.
Abstract Link: http://www.medifocus.com/abstracts.php?gid=NR013&ID=28123288

Go to http://www.medifocus.com/links/NR013/0718 for direct online access to the above Abstract Links.

10.

Neuropsychiatric symptoms, behavioural disorders, and quality of life in Parkinson's disease.

Authors:	Balestrino R; Martinez-Martin P
Institution:	Department of Neuroscience "Rita Levi Montalcini", University of Turin, Via Cherasco 15, 10124 Torino, Italy. Madrid, Spain. Electronic address: pmartinez@isciii.es.
Journal:	J Neurol Sci. 2017 Feb 15;373:173-178. doi: 10.1016/j.jns.2016.12.060. Epub 2016 Dec 28.
Abstract Link:	http://www.medifocus.com/abstracts.php?gid=NR013&ID=28131182

11.

Cognitive Rehabilitation in Parkinson's Disease: Is it Feasible?

Authors:	Biundo R; Weis L; Fiorenzato E; Antonini A
Institution:	Parkinson's Disease and Movement Disorders Unit, San Camillo Hospital IRCCS, Venice, Italy. Venice, Italy. Venice, Italy. Venice, Italy.
Journal:	Arch Clin Neuropsychol. 2017 Nov 1;32(7):840-860. doi: 10.1093/arclin/acx092.
Abstract Link:	http://www.medifocus.com/abstracts.php?gid=NR013&ID=28961738

Go to http://www.medifocus.com/links/NR013/0718 for direct online access to the above Abstract Links.

12.

Walking on four limbs: A systematic review of Nordic Walking in Parkinson disease.

Authors: Bombieri F; Schena F; Pellegrini B; Barone P; Tinazzi M; Erro R
Institution: Department of Neuroscience, Biomedicine and Movement Sciences, Universita di Verona, Verona, Italy. Verona, Verona, Italy. Verona, Verona, Italy; CeRiSM (Research Centre of Mountain Sport and Health), University of Verona, Rovereto, Italy. Surgery, Neuroscience Section, University of Salerno, Salerno, Italy. Verona, Verona, Italy. Electronic address: michele.tinazzi@univr.it. Surgery, Neuroscience Section, University of Salerno, Salerno, Italy; Sobell Department of Motor Neuroscience and Movement Disorders, University College London (UCL) Institute of Neurology, London, United Kingdom.
Journal: Parkinsonism Relat Disord. 2017 May;38:8-12. doi: 10.1016/j.parkreldis.2017.02.004. Epub 2017 Feb 6.
Abstract Link: http://www.medifocus.com/abstracts.php?gid=NR013&ID=28202374

13.

Pimavanserin: A Novel Antipsychotic for Parkinson's Disease Psychosis.

Authors: Bozymski KM; Lowe DK; Pasternak KM; Gatesman TL; Crouse EL
Institution: 1 Virginia Commonwealth University Health System/Medical College of Virginia Hospitals, Richmond, VA, USA. Hospitals, Richmond, VA, USA. Hospitals, Richmond, VA, USA. Hospitals, Richmond, VA, USA. Hospitals, Richmond, VA, USA.
Journal: Ann Pharmacother. 2017 Jun;51(6):479-487. doi: 10.1177/1060028017693029. Epub 2017 Feb 1.
Abstract Link: http://www.medifocus.com/abstracts.php?gid=NR013&ID=28375643

Go to http://www.medifocus.com/links/NR013/0718 for direct online access to the above Abstract Links.

14.

Parkinson's Disease and Its Effect on the Lower Urinary Tract: Evaluation of Complications and Treatment Strategies.

Authors: Brucker BM; Kalra S
Institution: Department of Urology, New York University Langone Medical Center, 150 East 32nd street second floor, New York, NY 10016, USA; Department of Obstetrics and Gynecology, New York University Langone Medical Center, 550 First Avenue, New York, NY 10016, USA. Electronic address: Benjamin.Brucker@nyumc.org. street second floor, New York, NY 10016, USA.
Journal: Urol Clin North Am. 2017 Aug;44(3):415-428. doi: 10.1016/j.ucl.2017.04.008.
Abstract Link: http://www.medifocus.com/abstracts.php?gid=NR013&ID=28716322

15.

Parkinson's Disease: From Pathogenesis to Pharmacogenomics.

Author: Cacabelos R
Institution: EuroEspes Biomedical Research Center, Institute of Medical Science and Genomic Medicine, 15165-Bergondo, Corunna, Spain. rcacabelos@euroespes.com.
Journal: Int J Mol Sci. 2017 Mar 4;18(3). pii: E551. doi: 10.3390/ijms18030551.
Abstract Link: http://www.medifocus.com/abstracts.php?gid=NR013&ID=28273839

Go to http://www.medifocus.com/links/NR013/0718 for direct online access to the above Abstract Links.

16.

Safinamide for the treatment of Parkinson's disease.

Authors: deSouza RM; Schapira A
Institution: a Department of Clinical Neurosciences , Institute of Neurology, University College London , London , UK. College London , London , UK.
Journal: Expert Opin Pharmacother. 2017 Jun;18(9):937-943. doi: 10.1080/14656566.2017.1329819. Epub 2017 May 23.
Abstract Link: http://www.medifocus.com/abstracts.php?gid=NR013&ID=28504022

17.

Current approaches to the treatment of Parkinson's Disease.

Authors: Ellis JM; Fell MJ
Institution: Department of Discovery Chemistry, Merck & Co., Inc., 33 Avenue Louis Pasteur, Boston, MA 02115, USA. Electronic address: michael_ellis@merck.com. Boston, MA 02115, USA.
Journal: Bioorg Med Chem Lett. 2017 Sep 15;27(18):4247-4255. doi: 10.1016/j.bmcl.2017.07.075. Epub 2017 Jul 29.
Abstract Link: http://www.medifocus.com/abstracts.php?gid=NR013&ID=28869077

Go to http://www.medifocus.com/links/NR013/0718 for direct online access to the above Abstract Links.

18.

Falls in Parkinson's disease: A complex and evolving picture.

Authors: Fasano A; Canning CG; Hausdorff JM; Lord S; Rochester L

Institution: Morton and Gloria Shulman Movement Disorders Centre and the Edmond J. Safra Program in Parkinson's Disease, Toronto Western Hospital, UHN, Division of Neurology, University of Toronto, Toronto, Ontario, Canada. Sydney, Australia. Tel Aviv Sourasky Medical Center, Tel Aviv, Israel. of Medicine, Tel Aviv University, Tel Aviv, Israel. University Medical Center, Chicago, Illinois, US. Newcastle upon Tyne, UK.

Journal: Mov Disord. 2017 Nov;32(11):1524-1536. doi: 10.1002/mds.27195. Epub 2017 Oct 25.

Abstract Link: http://www.medifocus.com/abstracts.php?gid=NR013&ID=29067726

19.

Neuroprotection and neurorestoration as experimental therapeutics for Parkinson's disease.

Authors: Francardo V; Schmitz Y; Sulzer D; Cenci MA

Institution: Basal Ganglia Pathophysiology Unit, Department of Experimental Medical Science, Lund University, Lund, Sweden. Electronic address: Veronica.Francardo@med.lu.se. Center: Division of Molecular Therapeutics, New York State Psychiatric Institute, New York 10032, NY, USA. Center: Division of Molecular Therapeutics, New York State Psychiatric Institute, New York 10032, NY, USA. Lund University, Lund, Sweden. Electronic address: Angela.Cenci_Nilsson@med.lu.se.

Journal: Exp Neurol. 2017 Dec;298(Pt B):137-147. doi: 10.1016/j.expneurol.2017.10.001. Epub 2017 Oct 5.

Abstract Link: http://www.medifocus.com/abstracts.php?gid=NR013&ID=28988910

Go to http://www.medifocus.com/links/NR013/0718 for direct online access to the above Abstract Links.

20.

Cognitive and Neuropsychiatric Features of Early Parkinson's Disease.

Authors: Getz SJ; Levin B
Institution: Department of Neurology, Division of Neuropsychology, University of Miami Miller School of Medicine, Miami, FL, USA. School of Medicine, Miami, FL, USA.
Journal: Arch Clin Neuropsychol. 2017 Nov 1;32(7):769-785. doi: 10.1093/arclin/acx091.
Abstract Link: http://www.medifocus.com/abstracts.php?gid=NR013&ID=29077803

21.

Deep Brain Stimulation Target Selection for Parkinson's Disease.

Authors: Honey CR; Hamani C; Kalia SK; Sankar T; Picillo M; Munhoz RP; Fasano A; Panisset M
Institution: 1Division of Neurosurgery,University of British Columbia,Vancouver,British Columbia. of Alberta,Edmonton,Alberta. Program in Parkinson's Disease,Toronto Western Hospital,University Health Network,Toronto,Ontario. Program in Parkinson's Disease,Toronto Western Hospital,University Health Network,Toronto,Ontario. Program in Parkinson's Disease,Toronto Western Hospital,University Health Network,Toronto,Ontario. Montreal Health Centre,Montreal,Quebec,Canada.
Journal: Can J Neurol Sci. 2017 Jan;44(1):3-8. doi: 10.1017/cjn.2016.22. Epub 2016 Mar 15.
Abstract Link: http://www.medifocus.com/abstracts.php?gid=NR013&ID=26976064

22.

Autophagy impairment in Parkinson's disease.

Authors: Karabiyik C; Lee MJ; Rubinsztein DC

Institution: Department of Medical Genetics, Cambridge Institute for Medical Research, Cambridge Biomedical Campus, Wellcome Trust/MRC Building, Cambridge Biomedical Campus, Hills Road, Cambridge CB2 0XY, U.K. College of Medicine, Seoul 03080, Korea dcr1000@cam.ac.uk minjlee@snu.ac.kr. Cambridge Biomedical Campus, Wellcome Trust/MRC Building, Cambridge Biomedical Campus, Hills Road, Cambridge CB2 0XY, U.K. dcr1000@cam.ac.uk minjlee@snu.ac.kr. Campus, Hills Road, Cambridge, U.K.

Journal: Essays Biochem. 2017 Dec 12;61(6):711-720. doi: 10.1042/EBC20170023. Print 2017 Dec 12.

Abstract Link: http://www.medifocus.com/abstracts.php?gid=NR013&ID=29233880

23.

A comprehensive overview of the neuropsychiatry of Parkinson's disease: A review.

Authors: Khan MA; Quadri SA; Tohid H

Institution: Dow Medical College, Dow University of Health Sciences, Karachi, Pakistan.

Journal: Bull Menninger Clin. 2017 Winter;81(1):53-105. doi: 10.1521/bumc.2017.81.1.53.

Abstract Link: http://www.medifocus.com/abstracts.php?gid=NR013&ID=28271905

Go to http://www.medifocus.com/links/NR013/0718 for direct online access to the above Abstract Links.

24.

Pimavanserin, a novel antipsychotic for management of Parkinson's disease psychosis.

Authors: Kianirad Y; Simuni T
Institution: a Department of Neurology , Northwestern University, Feinberg School of Medicine , Chicago , IL , USA. , Chicago , IL , USA.
Journal: Expert Rev Clin Pharmacol. 2017 Nov;10(11):1161-1168. doi: 10.1080/17512433.2017.1369405. Epub 2017 Oct 17.
Abstract Link: http://www.medifocus.com/abstracts.php?gid=NR013&ID=28817967

25.

Minimally invasive motor cortex stimulation for Parkinson's disease.

Authors: Lavano A; Guzzi G; DE Rose M; Romano M; Della Torre A; Vescio G; Deodato F; Lavano F; Volpentesta G
Institution: Department of Neurosurgery, "Magna Graecia" University, Catanzaro, Italy - lavano@unicz.it.
Journal: J Neurosurg Sci. 2017 Feb;61(1):77-87. Epub 2015 Apr 17.
Abstract Link: http://www.medifocus.com/abstracts.php?gid=NR013&ID=25881652

26.

A Meta-Analysis of Nonpharmacological Interventions for People With Parkinson's Disease.

Authors: Lee J; Choi M; Yoo Y
Institution: 1 Yonsei University, Seodaemun-gu, Seoul, Korea.
Journal: Clin Nurs Res. 2017 Oct;26(5):608-631. doi: 10.1177/1054773816655091. Epub 2016 Jun 17.
Abstract Link: http://www.medifocus.com/abstracts.php?gid=NR013&ID=27318243

Go to http://www.medifocus.com/links/NR013/0718 for direct online access to the above Abstract Links.

27.

Clinical effectiveness of acupuncture on Parkinson disease: A PRISMA-compliant systematic review and meta-analysis.

Authors: Lee SH; Lim S

Institution: aDepartment of Applied Korean Medicine, College of Korean Medicine, Graduate School, Kyung Hee University bResearch Group of Pain and Neuroscience, WHO Collaborating Center for Traditional Medicine, East-West Medical Research Institute cDepartment of Meridian and Acupoint, College of Korean Medicine, Kyung Hee University, Seoul, Republic of Korea.

Journal: Medicine (Baltimore). 2017 Jan;96(3):e5836. doi: 10.1097/MD.0000000000005836.

Abstract Link: http://www.medifocus.com/abstracts.php?gid=NR013&ID=28099340

28.

Management of lower urinary tract symptoms in Parkinson's disease in the neurology clinic.

Authors: Madan A; Ray S; Burdick D; Agarwal P

Institution: a College of Medical and Dental Sciences , University of Birmingham , Birmingham , UK. Kirkland , WA , USA. Kirkland , WA , USA. Kirkland , WA , USA.

Journal: Int J Neurosci. 2017 Dec;127(12):1136-1149. doi: 10.1080/00207454.2017.1327857. Epub 2017 May 25.

Abstract Link: http://www.medifocus.com/abstracts.php?gid=NR013&ID=28478699

Go to http://www.medifocus.com/links/NR013/0718 for direct online access to the above Abstract Links.

29.

Preclinical and Potential Applications of Common Western Herbal Supplements as Complementary Treatment in Parkinson's Disease.

Authors: Morgan LA; Grundmann O
Institution: a Department of Medicinal Chemistry , College of Pharmacy, University of Florida , Gainesville , FL , USA. , Gainesville , FL , USA.
Journal: J Diet Suppl. 2017 Jul 4;14(4):453-466. doi: 10.1080/19390211.2016.1263710. Epub 2017 Jan 17.
Abstract Link: http://www.medifocus.com/abstracts.php?gid=NR013&ID=28095073

30.

Clinical approaches to the development of a neuroprotective therapy for PD.

Authors: Olanow CW; Kieburtz K; Katz R
Institution: Clintrex LLC, United States; Dept of Neurology, Dept of Neuroscience, Mount Sinai School of Medicine, New York, NY, United States. Electronic address: Warren.olanow@mssm.edu. States. States.
Journal: Exp Neurol. 2017 Dec;298(Pt B):246-251. doi: 10.1016/j.expneurol.2017.06.018. Epub 2017 Jun 13.
Abstract Link: http://www.medifocus.com/abstracts.php?gid=NR013&ID=28622912

31.

Management of Parkinson's disease in Ayurveda: Medicinal plants and adjuvant measures.

Authors: Pathak-Gandhi N; Vaidya AD
Institution: Medical Research Centre - Kasturba Health Society, 17 K Desai Road, Mumbai, India. Electronic address: namyata@gmail.com. India. Electronic address: ashokdbv@gmail.com.
Journal: J Ethnopharmacol. 2017 Feb 2;197:46-51. doi: 10.1016/j.jep.2016.08.020. Epub 2016 Aug 17.
Abstract Link: http://www.medifocus.com/abstracts.php?gid=NR013&ID=27544001

Go to http://www.medifocus.com/links/NR013/0718 for direct online access to the above Abstract Links.

32.

Opicapone for the treatment of Parkinson's disease.

Authors: Rodrigues FB; Ferreira JJ

Institution: a Laboratory of Clinical Pharmacology and Therapeutics, Faculty of Medicine , University of Lisbon , Lisboa , Portugal. Medicine , University of Lisbon , Lisbon , Portugal. , London , UK. University of Lisbon , Lisboa , Portugal. Medicine , University of Lisbon , Lisbon , Portugal.

Journal: Expert Opin Pharmacother. 2017 Mar;18(4):445-453. doi: 10.1080/14656566.2017.1294683. Epub 2017 Feb 22.

Abstract Link: http://www.medifocus.com/abstracts.php?gid=NR013&ID=28234566

33.

Who Can Diagnose Parkinson's Disease First? Role of Pre-motor Symptoms.

Authors: Rodriguez-Violante M; Zeron-Martinez R; Cervantes-Arriaga A; Corona T

Institution: Unidad de Investigacion de Enfermedades Neurodegenerativas Clinicas, Instituto Nacional de Neurologia y Neurocirugia, Ciudad de Mexico, Mexico; Clinica de Trastornos del Movimiento, Instituto Nacional de Neurologia y Neurocirugia, Ciudad de Mexico, Mexico.; Unidad de Investigacion de Enfermedades Neurodegenerativas Clinicas, Instituto Nacional de Neurologia y Neurocirugia, Ciudad de Mexico, Mexico. Electronic address: coronav@unam.mx.

Journal: Arch Med Res. 2017 Apr;48(3):221-227. doi: 10.1016/j.arcmed.2017.08.005. Epub 2017 Sep 4.

Abstract Link: http://www.medifocus.com/abstracts.php?gid=NR013&ID=28882322

Go to http://www.medifocus.com/links/NR013/0718 for direct online access to the above Abstract Links.

34.

Non-motor features of Parkinson disease.

Authors: Schapira AHV; Chaudhuri KR; Jenner P
Institution: Department of Clinical Neurosciences, University College London (UCL) Institute of Neurology, Royal Free Campus, Rowland Hill Street, London NW3 2PF, UK. Hospital, King's College London, Camberwell Road, London SE5 9RS, UK. Faculty of Life Sciences and Medicine, King's College London, Newcomen Street, London SE1 1UL, UK.
Journal: Nat Rev Neurosci. 2017 Jul;18(7):435-450. doi: 10.1038/nrn.2017.62. Epub 2017 Jun 8.
Abstract Link: http://www.medifocus.com/abstracts.php?gid=NR013&ID=28592904

35.

Music-based interventions in neurological rehabilitation.

Authors: Sihvonen AJ; Sarkamo T; Leo V; Tervaniemi M; Altenmuller E; Soinila S
Institution: Faculty of Medicine, University of Turku, Turku, Finland; Cognitive Brain Research Unit, Department of Psychology and Logopedics, Faculty of Medicine, University of Helsinki, Finland. Electronic address: ajsihv@utu.fi. of Medicine, University of Helsinki, Finland. of Medicine, University of Helsinki, Finland. of Medicine, University of Helsinki, Finland; CICERO Learning, University of Helsinki, Finland. Drama Hannover, Hanover, Germany. Clinical Neurosciences, Turku University Hospital, Turku, Finland.
Journal: Lancet Neurol. 2017 Aug;16(8):648-660. doi: 10.1016/S1474-4422(17)30168-0. Epub 2017 Jun 26.
Abstract Link: http://www.medifocus.com/abstracts.php?gid=NR013&ID=28663005

Go to http://www.medifocus.com/links/NR013/0718 for direct online access to the above Abstract Links.

36.

Intrajejunal levodopa infusion therapy for Parkinson's disease: practical and pragmatic tips for successful maintenance of therapy.

Authors: Titova N; Ray Chaudhuri K
Institution: a Department of Neurology, Neurosurgery and Medical Genetics, Federal State Budgetary Educational Institution of Higher Education , 'N.I. Pirogov Russian National Research Medical University' of the Ministry of Healthcare of the Russian Federation , Moscow , Russia. Excellence , Kings College and Kings College Hospital , London , UK. London , UK.
Journal: Expert Rev Neurother. 2017 Jun;17(6):529-537. doi: 10.1080/14737175.2017.1317595. Epub 2017 Apr 17.
Abstract Link: http://www.medifocus.com/abstracts.php?gid=NR013&ID=28406336

37.

Some Clinically Useful Information that Neuropsychology Provides Patients, Carepartners, Neurologists, and Neurosurgeons About Deep Brain Stimulation for Parkinson's Disease.

Author: Troster AI
Institution: Department of Clinical Neuropsychology and Center for Neuromodulation, Barrow Neurological Institute, Phoenix, AZ, USA.
Journal: Arch Clin Neuropsychol. 2017 Nov 1;32(7):810-828. doi: 10.1093/arclin/acx090.
Abstract Link: http://www.medifocus.com/abstracts.php?gid=NR013&ID=29077802

Go to http://www.medifocus.com/links/NR013/0718 for direct online access to the above Abstract Links.

38.

Evidence-Based Review of Pharmacotherapy Used for Parkinson's Disease Psychosis.

Authors: Wilby KJ; Johnson EG; Johnson HE; Ensom MHH
Institution: 1 Qatar University, Doha, Qatar. Canada.
Journal: Ann Pharmacother. 2017 Aug;51(8):682-695. doi: 10.1177/1060028017703992. Epub 2017 Apr 6.
Abstract Link: http://www.medifocus.com/abstracts.php?gid=NR013&ID=28385039

39.

The significance of uric acid in the diagnosis and treatment of Parkinson disease: An updated systemic review.

Authors: Yu Z; Zhang S; Wang D; Fan M; Gao F; Sun W; Li Z; Li S
Institution: aDepartment of Acupuncture, China-Japan Friendship Hospital, Beijing bDepartment of Neurology, The Affiliated Hospital of Yangzhou University, Yangzhou University, Yangzhou, Jiangsu Province cDepartment of Orthopedics, Tumd Right Banner Hospital, Baotou City dDepartment of Orthopedics, China-Japan Friendship Hospital, Beijing, China.
Journal: Medicine (Baltimore). 2017 Nov;96(45):e8502. doi: 10.1097/MD.0000000000008502.
Abstract Link: http://www.medifocus.com/abstracts.php?gid=NR013&ID=29137045

Go to http://www.medifocus.com/links/NR013/0718 for direct online access to the above Abstract Links.

40.

Recent advances in discovery and development of natural products as source for anti-Parkinson's disease lead compounds.

Authors: Zhang H; Bai L; He J; Zhong L; Duan X; Ouyang L; Zhu Y; Wang T; Zhang Y; Shi J

Institution: Sichuan Academy of Medical Science & Sichuan Provincial People's Hospital, School of Medicine of University of Electronic Science and Technology of China, Chinese Academy of Sciences Sichuan Translational Medicine Research Hospital, Chengdu 610072, China. Electronic address: shijianyoude@126.com.; State Key Laboratory of Biotherapy & Cancer Center, West China Hospital, Sichuan University, Collaborative Innovation Center of Biotherapy, Chengdu 610041, China. Electronic address: yiwenzhang@scu.edu.cn.

Journal: Eur J Med Chem. 2017 Dec 1;141:257-272. doi: 10.1016/j.ejmech.2017.09.068. Epub 2017 Sep 30.

Abstract Link: http://www.medifocus.com/abstracts.php?gid=NR013&ID=29031072

41.

The efficacy and safety of coenzyme Q10 in Parkinson's disease: a meta-analysis of randomized controlled trials.

Authors: Zhu ZG; Sun MX; Zhang WL; Wang WW; Jin YM; Xie CL

Institution: Department of Neurology, The First Affiliated Hospital of Wenzhou Medical University, Wenzhou, 325000, China. University, Wenzhou, 35000, China. University, Wenzhou, 325000, China. Yuying Children's Hospital of Wenzhou Medical University, Wenzhou, 325027, China. Children's Hospital of Wenzhou Medical University, Wenzhou, 325027, China. 69365560@qq.com. University, Wenzhou, 325000, China. xiechenglong1987@sina.com.

Journal: Neurol Sci. 2017 Feb;38(2):215-224. doi: 10.1007/s10072-016-2757-9. Epub 2016 Nov 9.

Abstract Link: http://www.medifocus.com/abstracts.php?gid=NR013&ID=27830343

Go to http://www.medifocus.com/links/NR013/0718 for direct online access to the above Abstract Links.

42.

Efficacy of antidepressive medication for depression in Parkinson disease: a network meta-analysis.

Authors: Zhuo C; Xue R; Luo L; Ji F; Tian H; Qu H; Lin X; Jiang R; Tao R

Institution: aDepartment of Psychological Medicine, Wenzhou Seventh People's Hospital, Wenzhou, Zhejiang bInstitute of Mental Health, Jining Medical University, Jining, Shandong cDepartment of Psychological Medicine, Tianjin Mental Health Center dDepartment of Psychological Medicine, Tianjin Anning Hospital eDepartment of Neurology, Tianjin Medical University General Hospital, Tianjin fDepartment of Psychological Medicine, Chinese PLA (People's Liberation Army) General Hospital gDepartment of Psychological Medicine, General Hospital of Beijing Military Region, Chinese PLA, Beijing, China.

Journal: Medicine (Baltimore). 2017 Jun;96(22):e6698. doi: 10.1097/MD.0000000000006698.

Abstract Link: http://www.medifocus.com/abstracts.php?gid=NR013&ID=28562526

Go to http://www.medifocus.com/links/NR013/0718 for direct online access to the above Abstract Links.

43.

Parkinson's disease: Autoimmunity and neuroinflammation.

Authors: De Virgilio A; Greco A; Fabbrini G; Inghilleri M; Rizzo MI; Gallo A; Conte M; Rosato C; Ciniglio Appiani M; de Vincentiis M

Institution: Department Organs of Sense, ENT Section, 'Sapienza' University of Rome, Viale del Policlinico 155, 00100, Rome, Italy; Department of Surgical Science, 'Sapienza' University of Rome, Viale del Policlinico 155, 00100, Rome, Italy. Electronic address: mariaidarizzo@gmail.com.; Department Organs of Sense, ENT Section, 'Sapienza' University of Rome, Viale del Policlinico 155, 00100, Rome, Italy.; Department of Neurology and Psychiatry, 'Sapienza' University of Rome, Viale del Policlinico 155, 00100, Rome, Italy.; Department of Medico-Surgical Sciences and Biotechnologies, Otorhinolaryngology Section, 'Sapienza' University of Rome, Corso della Repubblica, 79, 04100 Latina, Italy.

Journal: Autoimmun Rev. 2016 Oct;15(10):1005-11. doi: 10.1016/j.autrev.2016.07.022. Epub 2016 Aug 4.

Abstract Link: http://www.medifocus.com/abstracts.php?gid=NR013&ID=27497913

44.

Advances in levodopa therapy for Parkinson disease: Review of RYTARY (carbidopa and levodopa) clinical efficacy and safety.

Authors: Dhall R; Kreitzman DL

Institution: From the Parkinson's Institute and Clinical Center (R.D.), Sunnyvale, CA; and Parkinson's Disease and Movement Disorder Center of Long Island (D.L.K.), Commack, NY. drdhall@gmail.com.

Journal: Neurology. 2016 Apr 5;86(14 Suppl 1):S13-24. doi: 10.1212/WNL.0000000000002510. Epub 2016 Apr 4.

Abstract Link: http://www.medifocus.com/abstracts.php?gid=NR013&ID=27044646

45.

Integrated Approach for Pain Management in Parkinson Disease.

Authors: Geroin C; Gandolfi M; Bruno V; Smania N; Tinazzi M
Institution: Neuromotor and Cognitive Rehabilitation Research Center (CRRNC), Department of Neurological, Biomedical and Movement Sciences, University of Verona, P.le L.A. Scuro 10, 37134, Verona, Italy. christian.geroin@univr.it. Neurological, Biomedical and Movement Sciences, University of Verona, P.le L.A. Scuro 10, 37134, Verona, Italy. marialuisa.gandolfi@univr.it. 10, 37134, Verona, Italy. marialuisa.gandolfi@univr.it. Program in Parkinson's Disease, Toronto Western Hospital, University Health Network, Toronto, ON, Canada. veubru@gmail.com. Neurological, Biomedical and Movement Sciences, University of Verona, P.le L.A. Scuro 10, 37134, Verona, Italy. nicola.smania@univr.it. 10, 37134, Verona, Italy. nicola.smania@univr.it. Biomedical and Movement Sciences, University of Verona, P.le Scuro 10, 37134, Verona, Italy. michele.tinazzi@univr.it.
Journal: Curr Neurol Neurosci Rep. 2016 Apr;16(4):28. doi: 10.1007/s11910-016-0628-7.
Abstract Link: http://www.medifocus.com/abstracts.php?gid=NR013&ID=26879763

46.

Lewy Body Dementias: Dementia With Lewy Bodies and Parkinson Disease Dementia.

Author: Gomperts SN
Journal: Continuum (Minneap Minn). 2016 Apr;22(2 Dementia):435-63. doi: 10.1212/CON.0000000000000309.
Abstract Link: http://www.medifocus.com/abstracts.php?gid=NR013&ID=27042903

Go to http://www.medifocus.com/links/NR013/0718 for direct online access to the above Abstract Links.

47.

Novel Approaches to Optimization of Levodopa Therapy for Parkinson's Disease.

Authors: Kianirad Y; Simuni T
Institution: Department of Neurology, Feinberg School of Medicine, Northwestern University, Chicago, IL, USA. Yasaman.Kianirad@northwestern.edu. Feinberg School of Medicine, Northwestern University, Abbott Hall 11th Floor, 710 North Lake Shore Drive, Chicago, IL, 60611, USA. TSimuni@nm.org.
Journal: Curr Neurol Neurosci Rep. 2016 Apr;16(4):34. doi: 10.1007/s11910-016-0635-8.
Abstract Link: http://www.medifocus.com/abstracts.php?gid=NR013&ID=26898686

48.

Levodopa therapy for Parkinson disease: A look backward and forward.

Authors: LeWitt PA; Fahn S
Institution: From the Department of Neurology (P.A.L.), Henry Ford Hospital; Department of Neurology (P.A.L.), Wayne State University School of Medicine, Detroit, MI; and Department of Neurology (S.F.), Columbia University Medical Center, New York, NY. plewitt1@hfhs.org.
Journal: Neurology. 2016 Apr 5;86(14 Suppl 1):S3-12. doi: 10.1212/WNL.0000000000002509. Epub 2016 Apr 4.
Abstract Link: http://www.medifocus.com/abstracts.php?gid=NR013&ID=27044648

49.

Clinical translation of stem cell transplantation in Parkinson's disease.

Author: Lindvall O
Institution: Laboratory of Stem Cells and Restorative Neurology, Lund Stem Cell Center, University Hospital, Lund, Sweden.
Journal: J Intern Med. 2016 Jan;279(1):30-40. doi: 10.1111/joim.12415. Epub 2015 Aug 31.
Abstract Link: http://www.medifocus.com/abstracts.php?gid=NR013&ID=26332959

Go to http://www.medifocus.com/links/NR013/0718 for direct online access to the above Abstract Links.

50.

The nonmotor features of Parkinson's disease: pathophysiology and management advances.

Authors: Reichmann H; Brandt MD; Klingelhoefer L
Institution: Department of Neurology, Technical University Dresden, Dresden, Germany.
Journal: Curr Opin Neurol. 2016 Aug;29(4):467-73. doi: 10.1097/WCO.0000000000000348.
Abstract Link: http://www.medifocus.com/abstracts.php?gid=NR013&ID=27262147

51.

Continuous dopaminergic stimulation therapy for Parkinson's disease - recent advances.

Authors: Timpka J; Mundt-Petersen U; Odin P
Institution: aDepartment of Clinical Sciences Lund, Faculty of Medicine, Lund University bDepartment of Neurology, Skane University Hospital, Lund, Sweden cDepartment of Neurology, Central Hospital, Bremerhaven, Germany.
Journal: Curr Opin Neurol. 2016 Aug;29(4):474-9. doi: 10.1097/WCO.0000000000000354.
Abstract Link: http://www.medifocus.com/abstracts.php?gid=NR013&ID=27272976

Go to http://www.medifocus.com/links/NR013/0718 for direct online access to the above Abstract Links.

52.

Emerging targets and new small molecule therapies in Parkinson's disease treatment.

Authors: Zhang H; Tong R; Bai L; Shi J; Ouyang L

Institution: Sichuan Academy of Medical Science & Sichuan Provincial People's Hospital, School of Medicine of University of Electronic Science and Technology of China, Chinese Academy of Sciences Sichuan Translational Medicine Research Hospital, Chengdu 610072, China.; Sichuan Academy of Medical Science & Sichuan Provincial People's Hospital, School of Medicine of University of Electronic Science and Technology of China, Chinese Academy of Sciences Sichuan Translational Medicine Research Hospital, Chengdu 610072, China; State Key Laboratory of Biotherapy & Cancer Center, West China Hospital, Sichuan University, and Collaborative Innovation Center of Biotherapy, Chengdu 610041, China. Electronic address: shijianyoude@126.com.; State Key Laboratory of Biotherapy & Cancer Center, West China Hospital, Sichuan University, and Collaborative Innovation Center of Biotherapy, Chengdu 610041, China. Electronic address: ouyangliang@scu.edu.cn.

Journal: Bioorg Med Chem. 2016 Apr 1;24(7):1419-30. doi: 10.1016/j.bmc.2016.02.030. Epub 2016 Feb 24.

Abstract Link: http://www.medifocus.com/abstracts.php?gid=NR013&ID=26935940

Go to http://www.medifocus.com/links/NR013/0718 for direct online access to the above Abstract Links.

53.

Improving outcomes of subthalamic nucleus deep brain stimulation in Parkinson's disease.

Authors: Bari AA; Fasano A; Munhoz RP; Lozano AM
Institution: a 1 Division of Neurosurgery, Department of Surgery, Toronto Western Hospital, Krembil Neuroscience Center, University of Toronto, Toronto, ON M5T 2S8, Canada.; b 2 Morton and Gloria Shulman Movement Disorders Clinic and the Edmond J. Safra Program in Parkinson's Disease, Toronto Western Hospital, UHN, Division of Neurology, University of Toronto, Toronto, ON M5T 2S8, Canada.
Journal: Expert Rev Neurother. 2015 Oct;15(10):1151-60. doi: 10.1586/14737175.2015.1081815. Epub 2015 Sep 17.
Abstract Link: http://www.medifocus.com/abstracts.php?gid=NR013&ID=26377740

54.

Neuroinflammation in the pathophysiology of Parkinson's disease and therapeutic evidence of anti-inflammatory drugs.

Authors: Bassani TB; Vital MA; Rauh LK
Institution: Pontificia Universidade Catolica do Parana, Curitiba, PR, Brazil. Brazil.
Journal: Arq Neuropsiquiatr. 2015 Jul;73(7):616-23. doi: 10.1590/0004-282X20150057.
Abstract Link: http://www.medifocus.com/abstracts.php?gid=NR013&ID=26200058

Go to http://www.medifocus.com/links/NR013/0718 for direct online access to the above Abstract Links.

55.

Interventions for fatigue in Parkinson's disease.

Authors: Elbers RG; Verhoef J; van Wegen EE; Berendse HW; Kwakkel G
Institution: Department of Physiotherapy, University of Applied Sciences Leiden, Zernikedreef 11, PO Box 382, Leiden, Netherlands, 2300 AJ.
Journal: Cochrane Database Syst Rev. 2015 Oct 8;(10):CD010925. doi: 10.1002/14651858.CD010925.pub2.
Abstract Link: http://www.medifocus.com/abstracts.php?gid=NR013&ID=26447539

56.

NEURODEGENERATION. Alzheimer's and Parkinson's diseases: The prion concept in relation to assembled Abeta, tau, and alpha-synuclein.

Author: Goedert M
Institution: Laboratory of Molecular Biology, Medical Research Council, Francis Crick Avenue, Cambridge CB2 0QH, UK. mg@mrc-lmb.cam.ac.uk.
Journal: Science. 2015 Aug 7;349(6248):1255555. doi: 10.1126/science.1255555.
Abstract Link: http://www.medifocus.com/abstracts.php?gid=NR013&ID=26250687

57.

Cognitive training in Parkinson disease: A systematic review and meta-analysis.

Authors: Leung IH; Walton CC; Hallock H; Lewis SJ; Valenzuela M; Lampit A
Institution: From the Regenerative Neuroscience Group (I.H.K.L., H.H., M.V., A.L.) and Parkinson's Disease Research Clinic (C.C.W., S.J.G.L.), Brain and Mind Centre, University of Sydney, Australia. amit.lampit@sydney.edu.au.
Journal: Neurology. 2015 Nov 24;85(21):1843-51. doi: 10.1212/WNL.0000000000002145. Epub 2015 Oct 30.
Abstract Link: http://www.medifocus.com/abstracts.php?gid=NR013&ID=26519540

Go to http://www.medifocus.com/links/NR013/0718 for direct online access to the above Abstract Links.

58.

Recognition and treatment of autonomic disturbances in Parkinson's disease.

Authors: Li K; Reichmann H; Ziemssen T
Institution: a 1 Center of Clinical Neuroscience, Technical University Dresden, Dresden, Germany.
Journal: Expert Rev Neurother. 2015 Oct;15(10):1189-203. doi: 10.1586/14737175.2015.1095093.
Abstract Link: http://www.medifocus.com/abstracts.php?gid=NR013&ID=26416396

59.

Argentine tango in Parkinson disease--a systematic review and meta-analysis.

Authors: Lotzke D; Ostermann T; Bussing A
Institution: Quality of Life, Spirituality and Coping, Institute of Integrative Medicine, Faculty of Health, University Witten/Herdecke, Herdecke, Germany. desiree.loetzke@uni-wh.de. Herdecke, Germany. desiree.loetzke@uni-wh.de. Herdecke, Germany. thomas.ostermann@uni-wh.de. Witten/Herdecke, Herdecke, Germany. thomas.ostermann@uni-wh.de. Faculty of Health, University Witten/Herdecke, Herdecke, Germany. arndt.buessing@uni-wh.de. Herdecke, Germany. arndt.buessing@uni-wh.de.
Journal: BMC Neurol. 2015 Nov 5;15:226. doi: 10.1186/s12883-015-0484-0.
Abstract Link: http://www.medifocus.com/abstracts.php?gid=NR013&ID=26542475

Go to http://www.medifocus.com/links/NR013/0718 for direct online access to the above Abstract Links.

60.

Biomarkers of Parkinson's disease: present and future.

Authors: Miller DB; O'Callaghan JP
Institution: Centers for Disease Control and Prevention, National Institute for Occupational Safety and Health, Morgantown, WV 26505. Electronic address: dum6@cdc.gov. Safety and Health, Morgantown, WV 26505. Electronic address: jdo5@cdc.gov.
Journal: Metabolism. 2015 Mar;64(3 Suppl 1):S40-6. doi: 10.1016/j.metabol.2014.10.030. Epub 2014 Oct 31.
Abstract Link: http://www.medifocus.com/abstracts.php?gid=NR013&ID=25510818

61.

Safinamide for symptoms of Parkinson's disease.

Author: Muller T
Institution: Department of Neurology, St. Joseph Hospital Berlin-Weissensee, Berlin, Germany. thomas.mueller@ruhr-uni-bochum.de.
Journal: Drugs Today (Barc). 2015 Nov;51(11):653-9. doi: 10.1358/dot.2015.51.11.2414529.
Abstract Link: http://www.medifocus.com/abstracts.php?gid=NR013&ID=26744740

62.

Treating non-motor symptoms of Parkinson's disease with transplantation of stem cells.

Authors: Pantcheva P; Reyes S; Hoover J; Kaelber S; Borlongan CV
Institution: a Center of Excellence for Aging and Brain Repair, Department of Neurosurgery and Brain Repair, University of South Florida College of Medicine, Tampa, FL, USA.
Journal: Expert Rev Neurother. 2015 Oct;15(10):1231-40. doi: 10.1586/14737175.2015.1091727. Epub 2015 Sep 22.
Abstract Link: http://www.medifocus.com/abstracts.php?gid=NR013&ID=26394528

Go to http://www.medifocus.com/links/NR013/0718 for direct online access to the above Abstract Links.

63.

Dance for people with Parkinson disease: what is the evidence telling us?

Authors: Shanahan J; Morris ME; Bhriain ON; Saunders J; Clifford AM
Institution: Faculty of Education and Health Sciences, Department of Clinical Therapies, University of Limerick, Limerick, Ireland. Electronic address: joanne.s@outlook.com. Bundoora, Victoria, Australia. and Dance, University of Limerick, Limerick, Ireland. Limerick, Limerick, Ireland. University of Limerick, Limerick, Ireland.
Journal: Arch Phys Med Rehabil. 2015 Jan;96(1):141-53. doi: 10.1016/j.apmr.2014.08.017. Epub 2014 Sep 16.
Abstract Link: http://www.medifocus.com/abstracts.php?gid=NR013&ID=25223491

64.

Retromer in Alzheimer disease, Parkinson disease and other neurological disorders.

Authors: Small SA; Petsko GA
Institution: Taub Institute for Research on Alzheimer's Disease and the Ageing Brain, Departments of Neurology, Radiology, and Psychiatry, Columbia University College of Physicians and Surgeons, New York, New York 10032, USA. Neurology and Feil Family Brain and Mind Research Institute, Weill Cornell Medical College, New York, New York 10065, USA.
Journal: Nat Rev Neurosci. 2015 Mar;16(3):126-32. doi: 10.1038/nrn3896. Epub 2015 Feb 11.
Abstract Link: http://www.medifocus.com/abstracts.php?gid=NR013&ID=25669742

Go to http://www.medifocus.com/links/NR013/0718 for direct online access to the above Abstract Links.

65.

The relevance of pre-motor symptoms in Parkinson's disease.

Authors: Visanji N; Marras C
Institution: a Toronto Western Hospital, Morton and Gloria Shulman Movement Disorders Centre, 399 Bathurst Street, Toronto, Ontario, Canada.
Journal: Expert Rev Neurother. 2015 Oct;15(10):1205-17. doi: 10.1586/14737175.2015.1083423. Epub 2015 Sep 1.
Abstract Link: http://www.medifocus.com/abstracts.php?gid=NR013&ID=26416397

66.

Insights from late-onset familial parkinsonism on the pathogenesis of idiopathic Parkinson's disease.

Authors: Volta M; Milnerwood AJ; Farrer MJ
Institution: Department of Medical Genetics, Centre for Applied Neurogenetics, Djavad Mowafaghian Centre for Brain Health, University of British Columbia, Vancouver, BC, Canada. Electronic address: mfarrer@can.ubc.ca.; Division of Neurology, Centre for Applied Neurogenetics, Djavad Mowafaghian Centre for Brain Health, University of British Columbia, Vancouver, BC, Canada.
Journal: Lancet Neurol. 2015 Oct;14(10):1054-64. doi: 10.1016/S1474-4422(15)00186-6.
Abstract Link: http://www.medifocus.com/abstracts.php?gid=NR013&ID=26376970

Go to http://www.medifocus.com/links/NR013/0718 for direct online access to the above Abstract Links.

67.

Efficacy and safety of cholinesterase inhibitors and memantine in cognitive impairment in Parkinson's disease, Parkinson's disease dementia, and dementia with Lewy bodies: systematic review with meta-analysis and trial sequential analysis.

Authors: Wang HF; Yu JT; Tang SW; Jiang T; Tan CC; Meng XF; Wang C; Tan MS; Tan L

Institution: Department of Neurology, Qingdao Municipal Hospital, Nanjing Medical University, Nanjing, China.; Department of Neurology, Qingdao Municipal Hospital, Nanjing Medical University, Nanjing, China Department of Neurology, Qingdao Municipal Hospital, School of Medicine, Qingdao University, Qingdao, China Department of Neurology, Qingdao Municipal Hospital, College of Medicine and Pharmaceutics, Ocean University of China, Qingdao, China.; Department of Epidemiology and Biostatistics, School of Public Health, Nanjing Medical University, Nanjing, China.; Department of Neurology, Qingdao Municipal Hospital, School of Medicine, Qingdao University, Qingdao, China.

Journal: J Neurol Neurosurg Psychiatry. 2015 Feb;86(2):135-43. doi: 10.1136/jnnp-2014-307659. Epub 2014 May 14.

Abstract Link: http://www.medifocus.com/abstracts.php?gid=NR013&ID=24828899

68.

Acupuncture for Parkinson's Disease: a review of clinical, animal, and functional Magnetic Resonance Imaging studies.

Author: Xiao D

Journal: J Tradit Chin Med. 2015 Dec;35(6):709-17.

Abstract Link: http://www.medifocus.com/abstracts.php?gid=NR013&ID=26742319

Go to http://www.medifocus.com/links/NR013/0718 for direct online access to the above Abstract Links.

General Interest Articles

69.

Cognitive impairment in Parkinson's disease, Alzheimer's dementia, and vascular dementia: the role of the clock-drawing test.

Authors: Allone C; Lo Buono V; Corallo F; Bonanno L; Palmeri R; Di Lorenzo G; Marra A; Bramanti P; Marino S
Institution: Department of Clinical Neurosciences and Neurobioimaging. Istituto di Ricovero e Cura a Carattere Scientifico, Centro Neurolesi 'Bonino-Pulejo' Messina, Messina, Italy.; Department of Biomedical and Dental Sciences and Morphological and Functional Imaging, University of Messina, Messina, Italy.
Journal: Psychogeriatrics. 2018 Mar;18(2):123-131. doi: 10.1111/psyg.12294. Epub 2018 Feb 7.
Abstract Link: http://www.medifocus.com/abstracts.php?gid=NR013&ID=29417704

70.

Early occurrence of inspiratory muscle weakness in Parkinson's disease.

Authors: Baille G; Perez T; Devos D; Deken V; Defebvre L; Moreau C
Institution: Department of Neurology and Movement Disorders, Lille University Medical Center, Lille, France. Lille, France. France. Lille, France.
Journal: PLoS One. 2018 Jan 12;13(1):e0190400. doi: 10.1371/journal.pone.0190400. eCollection 2018.
Abstract Link: http://www.medifocus.com/abstracts.php?gid=NR013&ID=29329328

Go to http://www.medifocus.com/links/NR013/0718 for direct online access to the above Abstract Links.

71.

The Risk of Traumatic Brain Injury Occurring Among Patients with Parkinson Disease: A 14-Year Population-Based Study.

Authors: Eric Nyam TT; Ho CH; Wang YL; Lim SW; Wang JJ; Chio CC; Kuo JR; Wang CC

Institution: Department of Neurosurgery, Chi Mei Medical Center, Tainan, Taiwan.; Department of Medical Research, Chi Mei Medical Center, Tainan, Taiwan; Department of Hospital and Health Care Administration, Chia Nan University of Pharmacy and Science, Tainan, Taiwan.; Department of Rehabilitation, Chi Mei Medical Center, Tainan, Taiwan.; Department of Neurosurgery, Chi Mei Medical Center, Chiali, Tainan, Taiwan; Department of Nursing, Min-Hwei College of Health Care Management, Tainan, Taiwan.; Department of Medical Research, Chi Mei Medical Center, Tainan, Taiwan.

Journal: World Neurosurg. 2018 May;113:e328-e335. doi: 10.1016/j.wneu.2018.02.027. Epub 2018 Feb 13.

Abstract Link: http://www.medifocus.com/abstracts.php?gid=NR013&ID=29452320

72.

Superselective Thalamotomy in the Most Lateral Part of the Ventralis Intermedius Nucleus for Controlling Essential and Parkinsonian Tremor.

Authors: Hirato M; Miyagishima T; Takahashi A; Yoshimoto Y

Institution: Department of Neurosurgery, Gunma University Graduate School of Medicine, Maebashi, Gunma, Japan. Electronic address: mfhirato@gunma-u.ac.jp. Maebashi, Gunma, Japan. Maebashi, Gunma, Japan.

Journal: World Neurosurg. 2018 Jan;109:e630-e641. doi: 10.1016/j.wneu.2017.10.042. Epub 2017 Oct 17.

Abstract Link: http://www.medifocus.com/abstracts.php?gid=NR013&ID=29054781

Go to http://www.medifocus.com/links/NR013/0718 for direct online access to the above Abstract Links.

73.

Are dementia with Lewy bodies and Parkinson's disease dementia the same disease?

Authors: Jellinger KA; Korczyn AD
Institution: Institute of Clinical Neurobiology, Alberichgasse 5/13, A-1150, Vienna, Austria. kurt.jellinger@univie.ac.at.
Journal: BMC Med. 2018 Mar 6;16(1):34. doi: 10.1186/s12916-018-1016-8.
Abstract Link: http://www.medifocus.com/abstracts.php?gid=NR013&ID=29510692

74.

Predictors of Mortality in Nondemented Patients With Parkinson Disease: Motor Symptoms Versus Nonmotor Symptoms.

Authors: Santos-Garcia D; Suarez-Castro E; Ernandez J; Exposito-Ruiz I; Tunas-Gesto C; Aneiros-Diaz M; de Deus-Fonticoba T; Lopez-Fernandez M; Nunez-Arias D
Institution: 1 Section of Neurology, Hospital Arquitecto Marcide/Hospital Naval, Complexo Hospitalario Universitario de Ferrol (CHUF), Ferrol, A Coruna, Spain.; 2 Department of Biochemistry and Molecular Biology, Boston University, Boston, MA, USA.; 3 Department of Psychiatry, Hospital Naval, Complexo Hospitalario Universitario de Ferrol (CHUF), Ferrol, A Coruna, Spain.
Journal: J Geriatr Psychiatry Neurol. 2018 Jan;31(1):19-26. doi: 10.1177/0891988717743589. Epub 2017 Nov 30.
Abstract Link: http://www.medifocus.com/abstracts.php?gid=NR013&ID=29191070

75.

Experiences of Persons With Parkinson's Disease Engaged in Group Therapeutic Singing.

Authors: Stegemoller EL; Hurt TR; O'Connor MC; Camp RD; Green CW; Pattee JC; Williams EK
Institution: Iowa State University.
Journal: J Music Ther. 2018 Jan 13;54(4):405-431. doi: 10.1093/jmt/thx012.
Abstract Link: http://www.medifocus.com/abstracts.php?gid=NR013&ID=29182746

Go to http://www.medifocus.com/links/NR013/0718 for direct online access to the above Abstract Links.

76.

Depression in Parkinson's disease: A case-control study.

Authors: Wu YH; Chen YH; Chang MH; Lin CH
Institution: Section of Neurology, Taichung Veterans General Hospital, Taichung, Taiwan. Taichung, Taiwan.
Journal: PLoS One. 2018 Feb 1;13(2):e0192050. doi: 10.1371/journal.pone.0192050. eCollection 2018.
Abstract Link: http://www.medifocus.com/abstracts.php?gid=NR013&ID=29390032

77.

Nonmotor symptoms in de novo Parkinson disease comparing to normal aging.

Authors: Bago Rozankovic P; Rozankovic M; Vucak Novosel L; Stojic M
Institution: Department of Neurology, University Hospital Dubrava, Avenija Gojka Suska 6, 10000 Zagreb, Croatia. Electronic address: petrabago@yahoo.com. 10000 Zagreb, Croatia. 10000 Zagreb, Croatia. 10000 Zagreb, Croatia.
Journal: Clin Neurol Neurosurg. 2017 Apr;155:7-11. doi: 10.1016/j.clineuro.2017.02.002. Epub 2017 Feb 11.
Abstract Link: http://www.medifocus.com/abstracts.php?gid=NR013&ID=28212928

Go to http://www.medifocus.com/links/NR013/0718 for direct online access to the above Abstract Links.

78.

Human Trials of Stem Cell-Derived Dopamine Neurons for Parkinson's Disease: Dawn of a New Era.

Authors: Barker RA; Parmar M; Studer L; Takahashi J
Institution: Department of Clinical Neuroscience and Cambridge Stem Cell Institute, Forvie Site, Cambridge CB2 0PY, UK. Lund Stem Cell Centre, Department of Experimental Medical Science, Lund University, 22184, Lund, Sweden. Electronic address: malin.parmar@med.lu.se. Cancer Center, New York, NY 10022, USA. Kyoto University, 606-8507, Kyoto, Japan.
Journal: Cell Stem Cell. 2017 Nov 2;21(5):569-573. doi: 10.1016/j.stem.2017.09.014.
Abstract Link: http://www.medifocus.com/abstracts.php?gid=NR013&ID=29100010

79.

Impulse control disorders in advanced Parkinson's disease with dyskinesia: The ALTHEA study.

Authors: Biundo R; Weis L; Abbruzzese G; Calandra-Buonaura G; Cortelli P; Jori MC; Lopiano L; Marconi R; Matinella A; Morgante F; Nicoletti A; Tamburini T; Tinazzi M; Zappia M; Vorovenci RJ; Antonini A
Institution: Parkinson and Movement Disorders Unit, IRCCS Hospital San Camillo, Venice, Italy. Child Health, University of Genoa Genoa, Italy. Bologna, Bologna, Italy. Bologna, Italy.
Journal: Mov Disord. 2017 Nov;32(11):1557-1565. doi: 10.1002/mds.27181. Epub 2017 Sep 27.
Abstract Link: http://www.medifocus.com/abstracts.php?gid=NR013&ID=28960475

Go to http://www.medifocus.com/links/NR013/0718 for direct online access to the above Abstract Links.

80.

More than just dancing: experiences of people with Parkinson's disease in a therapeutic dance program.

Authors: Bognar S; DeFaria AM; O'Dwyer C; Pankiw E; Simic Bogler J; Teixeira S; Nyhof-Young J; Evans C
Institution: a Department of Physical Therapy , University of Toronto , Toronto , Canada. , Canada.
Journal: Disabil Rehabil. 2017 Jun;39(11):1073-1078. doi: 10.1080/09638288.2016.1175037. Epub 2016 May 23.
Abstract Link: http://www.medifocus.com/abstracts.php?gid=NR013&ID=27216230

81.

Glitazone use associated with reduced risk of Parkinson's disease.

Authors: Brakedal B; Flones I; Reiter SF; Torkildsen O; Dolle C; Assmus J; Haugarvoll K; Tzoulis C
Institution: Department of Neurology, Haukeland University Hospital, Bergen, Norway.
Journal: Mov Disord. 2017 Nov;32(11):1594-1599. doi: 10.1002/mds.27128. Epub 2017 Sep 1.
Abstract Link: http://www.medifocus.com/abstracts.php?gid=NR013&ID=28861893

82.

Parkinson Disease and Melanoma: Confirming and Reexamining an Association.

Authors: Dalvin LA; Damento GM; Yawn BP; Abbott BA; Hodge DO; Pulido JS
Institution: Department of Ophthalmology, Mayo Clinic, Rochester, MN. Center, Rochester, MN. Jacksonville, FL. Medicine, Mayo Clinic, Rochester, MN. Electronic address: pulido.jose@mayo.edu.
Journal: Mayo Clin Proc. 2017 Jul;92(7):1070-1079. doi: 10.1016/j.mayocp.2017.03.014.
Abstract Link: http://www.medifocus.com/abstracts.php?gid=NR013&ID=28688464

Go to http://www.medifocus.com/links/NR013/0718 for direct online access to the above Abstract Links.

83.

Dance therapy improves motor and cognitive functions in patients with Parkinson's disease.

Authors: de Natale ER; Paulus KS; Aiello E; Sanna B; Manca A; Sotgiu G; Leali PT; Deriu F
Institution: Department of Biomedical Sciences, University of Sassari, Sassari, Italy. Italy. Sassari, Italy. Sassari, Italy. Sassari, Italy.
Journal: NeuroRehabilitation. 2017;40(1):141-144. doi: 10.3233/NRE-161399.
Abstract Link: http://www.medifocus.com/abstracts.php?gid=NR013&ID=27814308

84.

REM Sleep Behavior Disorder and Cognitive Impairment in Parkinson's Disease.

Authors: Jozwiak N; Postuma RB; Montplaisir J; Latreille V; Panisset M; Chouinard S; Bourgouin PA; Gagnon JF
Institution: Department of Psychology, Universite du Quebec a Montreal, Montreal, QC, Canada. Montreal, Montreal, QC, Canada. Montreal, Montreal, QC, Canada. de Montreal, Montreal, QC, Canada. de Montreal, Montreal, QC, Canada. Montreal, Montreal, QC, Canada. Montreal, Montreal, QC, Canada.
Journal: Sleep. 2017 Aug 1;40(8). pii: 3884498. doi: 10.1093/sleep/zsx101.
Abstract Link: http://www.medifocus.com/abstracts.php?gid=NR013&ID=28645156

85.

Tobacco Use, Oral Health, and Risk of Parkinson's Disease.

Authors: Liu Z; Roosaar A; Axell T; Ye W
Journal: Am J Epidemiol. 2017 Apr 1;185(7):538-545. doi: 10.1093/aje/kww146.
Abstract Link: http://www.medifocus.com/abstracts.php?gid=NR013&ID=28338925

Go to http://www.medifocus.com/links/NR013/0718 for direct online access to the above Abstract Links.

86.

Natural history of falls in an incident cohort of Parkinson's disease: early evolution, risk and protective features.

Authors: Lord S; Galna B; Yarnall AJ; Morris R; Coleman S; Burn D; Rochester L

Institution: Human Movement Science, Institute of Neuroscience, Newcastle University Institute for Aging, Newcastle University, Newcastle upon Tyne, NE4 5PL, UK. lynn.rochester@ncl.ac.uk.; NIHR Newcastle Biomedical Research Centre, Newcastle upon Tyne Hospitals NHS Foundation Trust and Newcastle University, Newcastle upon Tyne, UK. lynn.rochester@ncl.ac.uk.; School of Clinical Sciences, Auckland University of Technology, Auckland, New Zealand.; Newcastle upon Tyne Hospitals NHS Foundation Trust, Newcastle upon Tyne, UK. lynn.rochester@ncl.ac.uk.; UK and Industrial Statistics Research Unit, Newcastle University, Newcastle upon Tyne, UK.

Journal: J Neurol. 2017 Nov;264(11):2268-2276. doi: 10.1007/s00415-017-8620-y. Epub 2017 Sep 25.

Abstract Link: http://www.medifocus.com/abstracts.php?gid=NR013&ID=28948348

87.

More than constipation - bowel symptoms in Parkinson's disease and their connection to gut microbiota.

Authors: Mertsalmi TH; Aho VTE; Pereira PAB; Paulin L; Pekkonen E; Auvinen P; Scheperjans F

Institution: Department of Neurology, Helsinki University Hospital, Helsinki, Finland. Helsinki, Finland. Helsinki, Helsinki, Finland. Helsinki, Helsinki, Finland. Helsinki, Helsinki, Finland. Helsinki, Finland. Helsinki, Helsinki, Finland.

Journal: Eur J Neurol. 2017 Nov;24(11):1375-1383. doi: 10.1111/ene.13398. Epub 2017 Sep 11.

Abstract Link: http://www.medifocus.com/abstracts.php?gid=NR013&ID=28891262

Go to http://www.medifocus.com/links/NR013/0718 for direct online access to the above Abstract Links.

88.

Reduced cognitive function in patients with Parkinson disease and obstructive sleep apnea.

Authors: Mery VP; Gros P; Lafontaine AL; Robinson A; Benedetti A; Kimoff RJ; Kaminska M

Institution: From Clinica Alemana de Santiago (V.P.M.), Facultad de Medicina, Universidad del Desarrollo, Santiago, Chile; and Respiratory Division & Sleep Laboratory (P.G., A.R., R.J.K., M.K.), Montreal Neurological Hospital (A.-L.L.), Departments of Medicine and Epidemiology, Biostatistics & Occupational Health (A.B.), and Respiratory Epidemiology and Clinical Research Unit, Research Institute (A.B., M.K.), McGill University Health Centre, Montreal, Canada. vmery@alemana.cl.

Journal: Neurology. 2017 Mar 21;88(12):1120-1128. doi: 10.1212/WNL.0000000000003738. Epub 2017 Feb 22.

Abstract Link: http://www.medifocus.com/abstracts.php?gid=NR013&ID=28228566

89.

Factors influencing psychological well-being in patients with Parkinson's disease.

Authors: Nicoletti A; Mostile G; Stocchi F; Abbruzzese G; Ceravolo R; Cortelli P; D'Amelio M; De Pandis MF; Fabbrini G; Pacchetti C; Pezzoli G; Tessitore A; Canesi M; Zappia M

Institution: Department "G.F. Ingrassia", Section of Neurosciences, University of Catania, Catania, Italy. Catania, Italy. Genoa, Genoa, Italy. Italy. Palermo, Palermo, Italy. Institute, Cassino (FR), Italy. University of Rome, Rome, Italy. Institute C. Mondino, Pavia, Italy. Second University of Naples, Naples, Italy.

Journal: PLoS One. 2017 Dec 15;12(12):e0189682. doi: 10.1371/journal.pone.0189682. eCollection 2017.

Abstract Link: http://www.medifocus.com/abstracts.php?gid=NR013&ID=29244834

Go to http://www.medifocus.com/links/NR013/0718 for direct online access to the above Abstract Links.

90.

Natural course of mild cognitive impairment in Parkinson disease: A 5-year population-based study.

Authors: Pedersen KF; Larsen JP; Tysnes OB; Alves G

Institution: From the Norwegian Centre for Movement Disorders (K.F.P., G.A.); Department of Neurology (K.F.P., G.A.) and Memory Clinic (K.F.P., G.A.), Stavanger University Hospital; Network for Medical Sciences (J.P.L.), University of Stavanger; and Department of Neurology (O.-B.T.), Haukeland University Hospital, Bergen, Norway. pekf@sus.no.

Journal: Neurology. 2017 Feb 21;88(8):767-774. doi: 10.1212/WNL.0000000000003634. Epub 2017 Jan 20.

Abstract Link: http://www.medifocus.com/abstracts.php?gid=NR013&ID=28108638

91.

Comorbid conditions associated with Parkinson's disease: A longitudinal and comparative study with Alzheimer disease and control subjects.

Authors: Santos Garcia D; Suarez Castro E; Exposito I; de Deus T; Tunas C; Aneiros A; Lopez Fernandez M; Nunez Arias D; Bermudez Torres M

Institution: Section of Neurology, Complejo Hospitalario Universitario de Ferrol (CHUF), Hospital A. Marcide, Ferrol, A Coruna, Spain. Electronic address: diegosangar@yahoo.es.; Department of Psychiatry, Complejo Hospitalario Universitario de Ferrol (CHUF), Hospital Naval, Ferrol, A Coruna, Spain.; Department of Family Medicine, Complejo Hospitalario Universitario de Ferrol (CHUF), Ferrol, A Coruna, Spain.

Journal: J Neurol Sci. 2017 Feb 15;373:210-215. doi: 10.1016/j.jns.2016.12.046. Epub 2016 Dec 29.

Abstract Link: http://www.medifocus.com/abstracts.php?gid=NR013&ID=28131190

Go to http://www.medifocus.com/links/NR013/0718 for direct online access to the above Abstract Links.

92.

Longitudinal decline of driving safety in Parkinson disease.

Authors: Uc EY; Rizzo M; O'Shea AMJ; Anderson SW; Dawson JD
Institution: From the Departments of Neurology (E.Y.U., M.R., S.W.A.) and Biostatistics (A.M.J.O., J.D.D.), University of Iowa; Neurology Service (E.Y.U.) and Comprehensive Access and Delivery Research & Evaluation (A.M.J.O.), Veterans Affairs Medical Center, Iowa City, IA; and Department of Neurology (M.R.), University of Nebraska, Omaha. ergun-uc@uiowa.edu.
Journal: Neurology. 2017 Nov 7;89(19):1951-1958. doi: 10.1212/WNL.0000000000004629. Epub 2017 Oct 11.
Abstract Link: http://www.medifocus.com/abstracts.php?gid=NR013&ID=29021353

93.

Treatment of Fatigue in Parkinson Disease.

Authors: Elbers RG; Berendse HW; Kwakkel G
Institution: Department of Physiotherapy, University of Applied Sciences, Leiden, the Netherlands2Department of Rehabilitation Medicine, VU University Medical Center, Amsterdam, the Netherlands. Netherlands. the Netherlands.
Journal: JAMA. 2016 Jun 7;315(21):2340-1. doi: 10.1001/jama.2016.5260.
Abstract Link: http://www.medifocus.com/abstracts.php?gid=NR013&ID=27272586

94.

What daily activities increase the risk of falling in Parkinson patients? An analysis of the utility of the ABC-16 scale.

Authors: Foongsathaporn C; Panyakaew P; Jitkritsadakul O; Bhidayasiri R
Institution: Chulalongkorn Center of Excellence for Parkinson Disease & Related Disorders, Department of Medicine, Faculty of Medicine, Chulalongkorn University, King Chulalongkorn Memorial Hospital, Thai Red Cross Society, Bangkok, 10330, Thailand.; Chulalongkorn Center of Excellence for Parkinson Disease & Related Disorders, Department of Medicine, Faculty of Medicine, Chulalongkorn University, King Chulalongkorn Memorial Hospital, Thai Red Cross Society, Bangkok, 10330, Thailand; Department of Rehabilitation Medicine, Juntendo University, Tokyo, Japan. Electronic address: rbh@chulapd.org.
Journal: J Neurol Sci. 2016 May 15;364:183-7. doi: 10.1016/j.jns.2016.03.037. Epub 2016 Mar 25.
Abstract Link: http://www.medifocus.com/abstracts.php?gid=NR013&ID=27084242

95.

Fall-related activity avoidance in relation to a history of falls or near falls, fear of falling and disease severity in people with Parkinson's disease.

Authors: Kader M; Iwarsson S; Odin P; Nilsson MH
Institution: Department of Health Sciences, Lund University, PO Box 157, SE-221 00, Lund, Sweden. manzur.kader@med.lu.se. Sweden. Hospital, Lund, Sweden. Sweden.
Journal: BMC Neurol. 2016 Jun 2;16:84. doi: 10.1186/s12883-016-0612-5.
Abstract Link: http://www.medifocus.com/abstracts.php?gid=NR013&ID=27250988

Go to http://www.medifocus.com/links/NR013/0718 for direct online access to the above Abstract Links.

96.

Can Parkinson's disease be cured by stimulating neurogenesis?

Author: Foltynie T
Journal: J Clin Invest. 2015 Mar 2;125(3):978-80. doi: 10.1172/JCI80822. Epub 2015 Feb 17.
Abstract Link: http://www.medifocus.com/abstracts.php?gid=NR013&ID=25689259

97.

CSF biomarkers and clinical progression of Parkinson disease.

Authors: Hall S; Surova Y; Ohrfelt A; Zetterberg H; Lindqvist D; Hansson O
Institution: From the Department of Neurology (S.H., Y.S.) and Memory Clinic (O.H.), Skane University Hospital; Department of Clinical Sciences (S.H., Y.S., D.L., O.H.), Lund University; Department of Psychiatry and Neurochemistry (A.O., H.Z.), Institute of Neuroscience and Physiology, the Sahlgrenska Academy at the University of Gothenburg, Gothenburg and Molndal, Sweden; UCL Institute of Neurology (H.Z.), Queen Square, London, UK; and Psychiatry Skane (D.L.), Lund, Sweden. Sara.Hall@med.lu.se Oskar.Hansson@med.lu.se.
Journal: Neurology. 2015 Jan 6;84(1):57-63. doi: 10.1212/WNL.0000000000001098. Epub 2014 Nov 19.
Abstract Link: http://www.medifocus.com/abstracts.php?gid=NR013&ID=25411441

Go to http://www.medifocus.com/links/NR013/0718 for direct online access to the above Abstract Links.

98.

Association between cigarette smoking and Parkinson's disease: A meta-analysis.

Authors: Li X; Li W; Liu G; Shen X; Tang Y
Institution: Shanghai Key Laboratory of New Drug Design, School of Pharmacy, East China University of Science and Technology, 130 Meilong Road, Shanghai 200237, China; Shanghai Institute of Materia Medica, Chinese Academy of Sciences, 555 Zuchongzhi Road, Shanghai 201203, China.; Shanghai Key Laboratory of New Drug Design, School of Pharmacy, East China University of Science and Technology, 130 Meilong Road, Shanghai 200237, China. Electronic address: ytang234@ecust.edu.cn.
Journal: Arch Gerontol Geriatr. 2015 Nov-Dec;61(3):510-6. doi: 10.1016/j.archger.2015.08.004. Epub 2015 Aug 4.
Abstract Link: http://www.medifocus.com/abstracts.php?gid=NR013&ID=26272284

99.

Greater motor progression in patients with Parkinson disease who carry LRRK2 risk variants.

Authors: Oosterveld LP; Allen JC Jr; Ng EY; Seah SH; Tay KY; Au WL; Tan EK; Tan LC
Institution: From the Department of Neurology (L.P.O., E.Y.L.N., S.-H.S., K.-Y.T., W.-L.A., E.-K.T., L.C.S.T.), Parkinson's Disease and Movement Disorders Centre, USA National Parkinson Foundation Centre of Excellence, National Neuroscience Institute; and Duke-NUS Graduate Medical School (J.C.A., W.-L.A., E.-K.T., L.C.S.T.), Singapore. louis_tan@nni.com.sg.
Journal: Neurology. 2015 Sep 22;85(12):1039-42. doi: 10.1212/WNL.0000000000001953. Epub 2015 Aug 26.
Abstract Link: http://www.medifocus.com/abstracts.php?gid=NR013&ID=26311745

100.

Emotional Awareness, Relationship Quality, and Satisfaction in Patients With Parkinson's Disease and Their Spousal Caregivers.

Authors: Ricciardi L; Pomponi M; Demartini B; Ricciardi D; Morabito B; Bernabei R; Bentivoglio AR
Institution: *Sobell Department, UCL Institute of Neurology, Queen Square, London, UK; daggerDepartment of Geriatrics, Neuroscience and Orthopaedics, "Gemelli" Hospital, Catholic University of Sacred Heart (UCSC), Rome; double daggerCattedra di Psichiatria - Dipartimento di Scienze della Salute, Universita` degli Studi di Milano; and section signInstitute of Neurology, Catholic University of Sacred Heart, Rome, Italy.
Journal: J Nerv Ment Dis. 2015 Aug;203(8):646-9. doi: 10.1097/NMD.0000000000000342.
Abstract Link: http://www.medifocus.com/abstracts.php?gid=NR013&ID=26226241

101.

Treadmill Training Improves Forward and Backward Gait in Early Parkinson Disease.

Authors: Tseng IJ; Yuan RY; Jeng C
Institution: From the School of Gerontology Health Management, College of Nursing, Taipei Medical University (I-JT); Department of Neurology, Taipei Medical University Hospital (R-YY); and Department of Neurology, School of Medicine, College of Medicine (R-YY), and Graduate Institute of Nursing, College of Nursing (CJ), Taipei Medical University, Taipei, Taiwan.
Journal: Am J Phys Med Rehabil. 2015 Oct;94(10):811-9. doi: 10.1097/PHM.0000000000000273.
Abstract Link: http://www.medifocus.com/abstracts.php?gid=NR013&ID=25802958

Go to http://www.medifocus.com/links/NR013/0718 for direct online access to the above Abstract Links.

Drug Therapy Articles

102.

Comparison of the Efficacy of Different Drugs on Non-Motor Symptoms of Parkinson's Disease: a Network Meta-Analysis.

Authors: Li BD; Cui JJ; Song J; Qi C; Ma PF; Wang YR; Bai J
Institution: Department of Neurology, Hebei Province Cangzhou Hospital of Integrated Traditional and Western Medicine, Cangzhou, China.; Dongzhimen Hospital, Beijing University of Chinese Medicine, Beijing, China.
Journal: Cell Physiol Biochem. 2018;45(1):119-130. doi: 10.1159/000486252. Epub 2018 Jan 15.
Abstract Link: http://www.medifocus.com/abstracts.php?gid=NR013&ID=29339630

103.

Successful Use of Escitalopram for the Treatment of Visual Hallucinations in Patients With Parkinson Disease.

Authors: Bergman J; Lerner PP; Sokolik S; Lerner V; Kreinin A; Miodownik C
Institution: *Mental Health Center, Ma'ale Carmel, The Ruth and Bruce Rappaport Faculty of Medicine, Technion, Haifa; daggerGeha Mental Health Center, Petakh Tikva; double daggerIsrael Defense Force, Tel Aviv; and section signBe'er-Sheva Mental Health Center, Faculty of Health Sciences, Ben-Gurion University of the Negev, Be'er-Sheva, Israel.
Journal: Clin Neuropharmacol. 2017 Nov/Dec;40(6):246-250. doi: 10.1097/WNF.0000000000000254.
Abstract Link: http://www.medifocus.com/abstracts.php?gid=NR013&ID=29059136

104.

The cost-effectiveness of levodopa/carbidopa intestinal gel compared to standard care in advanced Parkinson's disease.

Authors: Lowin J; Sail K; Baj R; Jalundhwala YJ; Marshall TS; Konwea H; Chaudhuri KR
Institution: a QuintilesIMS , London , UK.
Journal: J Med Econ. 2017 Nov;20(11):1207-1215. doi: 10.1080/13696998.2017.1379411. Epub 2017 Sep 21.
Abstract Link: http://www.medifocus.com/abstracts.php?gid=NR013&ID=28895769

105.

Switching L-dopa Therapy from Pulsatile to Pulse Administration Reduces Motor Complications in Parkinson's Disease.

Authors: Mostile G; Nicoletti A; Dibilio V; Luca A; Raciti L; Sciacca G; Cicero CE; Vasta R; Donzuso G; Contrafatto D; Zappia M
Institution: Dipartimento "G.F. Ingrassia", Sezione di Neuroscienze, Universita Degli Studi di Catania, Catania, Italy.
Journal: Clin Neuropharmacol. 2017 Jan/Feb;40(1):6-10. doi: 10.1097/WNF.0000000000000186.
Abstract Link: http://www.medifocus.com/abstracts.php?gid=NR013&ID=27879548

106.

First clinical experience with levodopa/carbidopa microtablets in Parkinson's disease.

Authors: Senek M; Hellstrom M; Albo J; Svenningsson P; Nyholm D
Institution: Department of Neuroscience, Neurology, Uppsala University, Uppsala, Sweden.
Journal: Acta Neurol Scand. 2017 Dec;136(6):727-731. doi: 10.1111/ane.12756. Epub 2017 Mar 15.
Abstract Link: http://www.medifocus.com/abstracts.php?gid=NR013&ID=28299787

Go to http://www.medifocus.com/links/NR013/0718 for direct online access to the above Abstract Links.

107.

Chinese medicine for idiopathic Parkinson's disease: A meta analysis of randomized controlled trials.

Authors: Wei W; Chen HY; Fan W; Ye SF; Xu YH; Cai J
Institution: College of Integrative Medicine, Fujian University of Traditional Chinese Medicine, Fuzhou, 350122, China. 441000, China. Province, 364000, China. Fuzhou, 350003, China. Medicine, Fuzhou, 350122, China. caij1@163.com.
Journal: Chin J Integr Med. 2017 Jan;23(1):55-61. doi: 10.1007/s11655-016-2618-7. Epub 2016 Oct 27.
Abstract Link: http://www.medifocus.com/abstracts.php?gid=NR013&ID=27796824

108.

The Efficacy of Istradefylline for Treating Mild Wearing-Off in Parkinson Disease.

Authors: Yabe I; Kitagawa M; Takahashi I; Matsushima M; Sasaki H
Institution: *Department of Neurology, Faculty of Medicine and Graduate School of Medicine, Hokkaido University; and daggerDepartment of Neurology, Sapporo Teishinkai Hospital, Sapporo, Japan.
Journal: Clin Neuropharmacol. 2017 Nov/Dec;40(6):261-263. doi: 10.1097/WNF.0000000000000249.
Abstract Link: http://www.medifocus.com/abstracts.php?gid=NR013&ID=28976411

Go to http://www.medifocus.com/links/NR013/0718 for direct online access to the above Abstract Links.

109.

What to do when people with Parkinson's disease cannot take their usual oral medications.

Authors: Alty J; Robson J; Duggan-Carter P; Jamieson S
Institution: Department of Neurosciences, Leeds Teaching Hospitals NHS Trust, Leeds, West Yorkshire, UK University of Leeds Hull York Medical School, University of York. Yorkshire, UK. Yorkshire, UK. Yorkshire, UK University of Leeds Hull York Medical School, University of York.
Journal: Pract Neurol. 2016 Apr;16(2):122-8. doi: 10.1136/practneurol-2015-001267. Epub 2015 Dec 30.
Abstract Link: http://www.medifocus.com/abstracts.php?gid=NR013&ID=26719485

110.

Physicians' experience with RYTARY (carbidopa and levodopa) extended-release capsules in patients who have Parkinson disease.

Authors: Silver DE; Trosch RM
Institution: From the Coastal Neurological Medical Group, Inc. (D.E.S.), La Jolla, CA; and the Parkinson's and Movement Disorders Center (R.M.T.), Farmington Hills, MI. richardtrosch@comcast.net.
Journal: Neurology. 2016 Apr 5;86(14 Suppl 1):S25-35. doi: 10.1212/WNL.0000000000002511. Epub 2016 Apr 4.
Abstract Link: http://www.medifocus.com/abstracts.php?gid=NR013&ID=27044647

111.

Parkinson's disease: initial treatment of motor disorders.

Author:
Journal: Prescrire Int. 2015 Sep;24(163):215-7.
Abstract Link: http://www.medifocus.com/abstracts.php?gid=NR013&ID=26417634

Go to http://www.medifocus.com/links/NR013/0718 for direct online access to the above Abstract Links.

112.

Parkinson disease: Laying the foundations for disease-modifying therapies in PD.

Authors: Brundin P; Wyse R
Institution: Van Andel Research Institute, Translational Parkinson's Disease Research, Center for Neurodegenerative Science, 333 Bostwick Avenue NE, Grand Rapids, MI 49503, USA.
Journal: Nat Rev Neurol. 2015 Oct;11(10):553-5. doi: 10.1038/nrneurol.2015.150. Epub 2015 Aug 25.
Abstract Link: http://www.medifocus.com/abstracts.php?gid=NR013&ID=26303855

113.

Novel arylalkenylpropargylamines as neuroprotective, potent, and selective monoamine oxidase B inhibitors for the treatment of Parkinson's disease.

Authors: Huleatt PB; Khoo ML; Chua YY; Tan TW; Liew RS; Balogh B; Deme R; Goloncser F; Magyar K; Sheela DP; Ho HK; Sperlagh B; Matyus P; Chai CL
Institution: Institute of Chemical and Engineering Sciences , A* STAR (Agency of Science, Technology and Research), 8 Biomedical Grove, Neuros #07-01, Singapore 138665, Singapore.
Journal: J Med Chem. 2015 Feb 12;58(3):1400-19. doi: 10.1021/jm501722s. Epub 2015 Jan 28.
Abstract Link: http://www.medifocus.com/abstracts.php?gid=NR013&ID=25627172

Clinical Trials Articles

114.

Efficacy of Combined Treatment with Acupuncture and Bee Venom Acupuncture as an Adjunctive Treatment for Parkinson's Disease.

Authors:	Cho SY; Lee YE; Doo KH; Lee JH; Jung WS; Moon SK; Park JM; Ko CN; Kim H; Rhee HY; Park HJ; Park SU
Institution:	1 Department of Cardiology and Neurology, College of Korean Medicine, Kyung Hee University , Seoul, Republic of Korea.; 2 Stroke and Neurological Disorders Center, Kyung Hee University Hospital at Gangdong , Seoul, Republic of Korea.; 3 Department of Epidemiology and Biostatistics, Graduate School of Public Health and Institute of Health and Environment, Seoul University , Seoul, Republic of Korea.; 4 Department of Neurology, Kyung Hee University Hospital at Gangdong, College of Medicine, Kyung Hee University , Seoul, Republic of Korea.; 5 Integrative Parkinson's Disease Research Group, Acupuncture and Meridian Science Research Center, Kyung Hee University , Seoul, Republic of Korea.
Journal:	J Altern Complement Med. 2018 Jan;24(1):25-32. doi: 10.1089/acm.2016.0250. Epub 2017 Jul 28.
Abstract Link:	http://www.medifocus.com/abstracts.php?gid=NR013&ID=28753030

115.

Acupuncture as Adjuvant Therapy for Sleep Disorders in Parkinson's Disease.

Authors:	Aroxa FH; Gondim IT; Santos EL; Coriolano MD; Asano AG; Asano NM
Institution:	Academic of Medicine graduation of Federal University of Pernambuco - Recife, Pernambuco (PE), Brazil. Recife (PE), Brazil. Recife (PE), Brazil. Recife (PE), Brazil. Recife (PE), Brazil. Brazil. Electronic address: nadjaasano@gmail.com.
Journal:	J Acupunct Meridian Stud. 2017 Jan;10(1):33-38. doi: 10.1016/j.jams.2016.12.007. Epub 2017 Jan 11.
Abstract Link:	http://www.medifocus.com/abstracts.php?gid=NR013&ID=28254099

Go to http://www.medifocus.com/links/NR013/0718 for direct online access to the above Abstract Links.

116.

Medical Cannabis in Parkinson Disease: Real-Life Patients' Experience.

Authors: Balash Y; Bar-Lev Schleider L; Korczyn AD; Shabtai H; Knaani J; Rosenberg A; Baruch Y; Djaldetti R; Giladi N; Gurevich T

Institution: *Movement Disorders Unit, Neurological Institute, Tel Aviv Sourasky Medical Center, Tel Aviv; daggerSackler School of Medicine, Tel Aviv University, Tel Aviv; double daggerTikun Olam, Research Department, Tel Aviv; section signSchool of Public Health, Epidemiology, Sackler School of Medicine, Tel-Aviv University, Tel-Aviv; parallelOneWorld Cannabis Ltd, Petah-Tikva; paragraph signMovement Disorders Center, Rabin Medical Center, Petah-Tikva; and #Sagol School of Neuroscience, Tel Aviv University, Tel Aviv, Israel.

Journal: Clin Neuropharmacol. 2017 Nov/Dec;40(6):268-272. doi: 10.1097/WNF.0000000000000246.

Abstract Link: http://www.medifocus.com/abstracts.php?gid=NR013&ID=29059132

117.

Safety and Efficacy of Focused Ultrasound Thalamotomy for Patients With Medication-Refractory, Tremor-Dominant Parkinson Disease: A Randomized Clinical Trial.

Authors: Bond AE; Shah BB; Huss DS; Dallapiazza RF; Warren A; Harrison MB; Sperling SA; Wang XQ; Gwinn R; Witt J; Ro S; Elias WJ

Institution: Department of Neurosurgery, University of Virginia Health Science Center, Charlottesville. Charlottesville. Charlottesville. Charlottesville. Charlottesville. Charlottesville. Charlottesville. Center, Charlottesville. Charlottesville.

Journal: JAMA Neurol. 2017 Dec 1;74(12):1412-1418. doi: 10.1001/jamaneurol.2017.3098.

Abstract Link: http://www.medifocus.com/abstracts.php?gid=NR013&ID=29084313

Go to http://www.medifocus.com/links/NR013/0718 for direct online access to the above Abstract Links.

118.

Benefits of Exercise on the Executive Functions in People with Parkinson Disease: A Controlled Clinical Trial.

Authors: de Oliveira RT; Felippe LA; Bucken Gobbi LT; Barbieri FA; Christofoletti G

Institution: From the Graduate Program in Health and Development, Universidade Federal de Mato Grosso do Sul, UFMS, Campo Grande, Mato Grosso do Sul (RTO, LAF, GC); Universidade Estadual Paulista, UNESP, Rio Claro (LTBG, FAB); and Universidade Estadual Paulista, UNESP, Bauru, Sao Paulo, Brazil (FAB).

Journal: Am J Phys Med Rehabil. 2017 May;96(5):301-306. doi: 10.1097/PHM.0000000000000612.

Abstract Link: http://www.medifocus.com/abstracts.php?gid=NR013&ID=27584142

119.

Osteopathic manipulation as a complementary approach to Parkinson's disease: A controlled pilot study.

Authors: DiFrancisco-Donoghue J; Apoznanski T; de Vries K; Jung MK; Mancini J; Yao S

Institution: Department of Osteopathic Medicine, College of Osteopathic Medicine, New York Institute of Technology (NYITCOM), Old Westbury, NY, USA. Westbury, NY, USA. Westbury, NY, USA. USA. Institute of Technology (NYITCOM), Old Westbury, NY, USA. Institute of Technology (NYITCOM), Old Westbury, NY, USA.

Journal: NeuroRehabilitation. 2017;40(1):145-151. doi: 10.3233/NRE-161400.

Abstract Link: http://www.medifocus.com/abstracts.php?gid=NR013&ID=27814309

Go to http://www.medifocus.com/links/NR013/0718 for direct online access to the above Abstract Links.

120.

Risk factors for early psychosis in PD: insights from the Parkinson's Progression Markers Initiative.

Authors: Ffytche DH; Pereira JB; Ballard C; Chaudhuri KR; Weintraub D; Aarsland D

Institution: KCL-PARCOG Group, Institute of Psychiatry, Psychology and Neuroscience, King's College London, London, UK.; Department of Old Age Psychiatry, Institute of Psychiatry, Psychology and Neuroscience, King's College London, London, UK.; Department of Neurobiology, Care Sciences and Society, Karolinska Institute, Stockholm, Sweden.; University of Exeter Medical School, University of Exeter, Exeter, Devon, UK.; Department of Basic and Clinical Neuroscience, The Maurice Wohl Clinical Neuroscience Institute, King's College London, London, UK.

Journal: J Neurol Neurosurg Psychiatry. 2017 Apr;88(4):325-331. doi: 10.1136/jnnp-2016-314832.

Abstract Link: http://www.medifocus.com/abstracts.php?gid=NR013&ID=28315846

121.

Cognitive Effects of Rasagiline in Mild-to-Moderate Stage Parkinson's Disease Without Dementia.

Authors: Frakey LL; Friedman JH

Institution: From the Memorial Hospital of Rhode Island-Medical Rehabilitation, Pawtucket, R.I. (LLF); and the Alpert Medical School of Brown University, Providence, R.I. (JHF).

Journal: J Neuropsychiatry Clin Neurosci. 2017 Winter;29(1):22-25. doi: 10.1176/appi.neuropsych.15050118. Epub 2016 Nov 10.

Abstract Link: http://www.medifocus.com/abstracts.php?gid=NR013&ID=27829318

Go to http://www.medifocus.com/links/NR013/0718 for direct online access to the above Abstract Links.

122.

A Phase Ib Randomized Controlled Study to Evaluate the Effectiveness of a Single-Dose of the NR2B Selective N-Methyl-D-Aspartate Antagonist MK-0657 on Levodopa-Induced Dyskinesias and Motor Symptoms in Patients With Parkinson Disease.

Authors: Herring WJ; Assaid C; Budd K; Vargo R; Mazenko RS; Lines C; Ellenbogen A; Verhagen Metman L
Institution: *Merck & Co, Inc, Kenilworth, NJ; daggerQUEST Research Institute, Bingham Farms, MI; and double daggerRush University Medical Center, Chicago, IL.
Journal: Clin Neuropharmacol. 2017 Nov/Dec;40(6):255-260. doi: 10.1097/WNF.0000000000000241.
Abstract Link: http://www.medifocus.com/abstracts.php?gid=NR013&ID=29059133

123.

Opicapone as Adjunct to Levodopa Therapy in Patients With Parkinson Disease and Motor Fluctuations: A Randomized Clinical Trial.

Authors: Lees AJ; Ferreira J; Rascol O; Poewe W; Rocha JF; McCrory M; Soares-da-Silva P
Institution: Reta Lila Weston Institute, University College London, London, England. Recherche Medicale (INSERM) and University Hospital of Toulouse, Toulouse, France4Department of Neurosciences, INSERM and University Hospital of Toulouse, Toulouse, France. Coronado, Portugal. Coronado, Portugal8Department of Pharmacology and Therapeutics, University Porto, Porto, Portugal.
Journal: JAMA Neurol. 2017 Feb 1;74(2):197-206. doi: 10.1001/jamaneurol.2016.4703.
Abstract Link: http://www.medifocus.com/abstracts.php?gid=NR013&ID=28027332

Go to http://www.medifocus.com/links/NR013/0718 for direct online access to the above Abstract Links.

124.

Remotely Programmed Deep Brain Stimulation of the Bilateral Subthalamic Nucleus for the Treatment of Primary Parkinson Disease: A Randomized Controlled Trial Investigating the Safety and Efficacy of a Novel Deep Brain Stimulation System.

Authors: Li D; Zhang C; Gault J; Wang W; Liu J; Shao M; Zhao Y; Zeljic K; Gao G; Sun B

Institution: Department of Functional Neurosurgery, Ruijin Hospital, Shanghai Jiao Tong University School of Medicine, Shanghai, China.

Journal: Stereotact Funct Neurosurg. 2017;95(3):174-182. doi: 10.1159/000475765. Epub 2017 Jun 2.

Abstract Link: http://www.medifocus.com/abstracts.php?gid=NR013&ID=28571034

Go to http://www.medifocus.com/links/NR013/0718 for direct online access to the above Abstract Links.

125.

Clinical manifestations of nonmotor symptoms in 1021 Japanese Parkinson's disease patients from 35 medical centers.

Authors: Maeda T; Shimo Y; Chiu SW; Yamaguchi T; Kashihara K; Tsuboi Y; Nomoto M; Hattori N; Watanabe H; Saiki H

Institution: Division of Neurology and Gerontology, Department of Internal Medicine, School of Medicine, Iwate Medical University, 19-1 Uchimaru, Morioka, Iwate 020-8505, Japan; Department of Neurology and Movement Disorder Research, Research Institute for Brain and Blood Vessels-Akita, 6-10 Senshukubotamachi, Akita 010-0874, Japan. Electronic address: maeda@iwate-med.ac.jp.; Department of Neurology, Juntendo University School of Medicine 3-1-3 Hongo, Bunkyo-ku, Tokyo 113-8431, Japan. Electronic address: yshimo@juntendo.ac.jp.; Division of Biostatistics, Tohoku University Graduate School of Medicine, 2-1 Seiryo-machi, Aoba-ku, Sendai, Miyagi, 980-8575, Japan. Electronic address: chiu@med.tohoku.ac.jp.; Division of Biostatistics, Tohoku University Graduate School of Medicine, 2-1 Seiryo-machi, Aoba-ku, Sendai, Miyagi, 980-8575, Japan. Electronic address: yamaguchi@med.tohoku.ac.jp.; Department of Neurology, Okayama Kyokuto Hospital, 567-1 Kurata, Okayama, 703-8265, Japan. Electronic address: kkashi@kyokuto.or.jp.

Journal: Parkinsonism Relat Disord. 2017 May;38:54-60. doi: 10.1016/j.parkreldis.2017.02.024. Epub 2017 Feb 21.

Abstract Link: http://www.medifocus.com/abstracts.php?gid=NR013&ID=28279596

126.

Botulinum Toxin in Parkinson Disease Tremor: A Randomized, Double-Blind, Placebo-Controlled Study With a Customized Injection Approach.

Authors: Mittal SO; Machado D; Richardson D; Dubey D; Jabbari B

Institution: Department of Neurology, Mayo Clinic, Rochester, MN. Electronic address: shivamommittal@gmail.com.

Journal: Mayo Clin Proc. 2017 Sep;92(9):1359-1367. doi: 10.1016/j.mayocp.2017.06.010. Epub 2017 Aug 5.

Abstract Link: http://www.medifocus.com/abstracts.php?gid=NR013&ID=28789780

Go to http://www.medifocus.com/links/NR013/0718 for direct online access to the above Abstract Links.

127.

Land Plus Aquatic Therapy Versus Land-Based Rehabilitation Alone for the Treatment of Balance Dysfunction in Parkinson Disease: A Randomized Controlled Study With 6-Month Follow-Up.

Authors: Palamara G; Gotti F; Maestri R; Bera R; Gargantini R; Bossio F; Zivi I; Volpe D; Ferrazzoli D; Frazzitta G

Institution: Department of Parkinson Disease and Brain Injury Rehabilitation, 'Moriggia-Pelascini' Hospital, Gravedona ed Uniti, Italy. Electronic address: grazia.palamara@gmail.com.; Department of Biomedical Engineering, Scientific Institute of Montescano, S. Maugeri Foundation IRCCS, Montescano, Italy.; Department of Physical Medicine and Rehabilitation, S. Raffaele Arcangelo Fatebenefratelli Hospital, Venice, Italy.

Journal: Arch Phys Med Rehabil. 2017 Jun;98(6):1077-1085. doi: 10.1016/j.apmr.2017.01.025. Epub 2017 Feb 27.

Abstract Link: http://www.medifocus.com/abstracts.php?gid=NR013&ID=28254636

Go to http://www.medifocus.com/links/NR013/0718 for direct online access to the above Abstract Links.

128.

Caffeine as symptomatic treatment for Parkinson disease (Cafe-PD): A randomized trial.

Authors: Postuma RB; Anang J; Pelletier A; Joseph L; Moscovich M; Grimes D; Furtado S; Munhoz RP; Appel-Cresswell S; Moro A; Borys A; Hobson D; Lang AE

Institution: From the Department of Neurology, Montreal General Hospital (R.B.P., A.P.), and Department of Epidemiology and Biostatistics (L.J.), McGill University, Montreal; Department of Neurology (J.A., A.B., D.H.), University of Manitoba, Winnipeg, Canada; Pontifical Catholic University of Parana (M.M., A.M.), Curitiba, Brazil; Department of Neurology (D.G.), Ottawa Hospital, University of Ottawa Brain and Mind Research Institute; Department of Neurology (S.F.), University of Calgary; Division of Neurology (R.P.M., A.E.L.), Toronto Western Hospital; and Department of Medicine, Division of Neurology, Djavad Mowafaghian Centre for Brain Health, and Pacific Parkinson's Research Centre (S.A.-C.), University of British Columbia, Vancouver, Canada. ron.postuma@mcgill.ca.

Journal: Neurology. 2017 Oct 24;89(17):1795-1803. doi: 10.1212/WNL.0000000000004568. Epub 2017 Sep 27.

Abstract Link: http://www.medifocus.com/abstracts.php?gid=NR013&ID=28954882

129.

Long-term tremor therapy for Parkinson and essential tremor with sensor-guided botulinum toxin type A injections.

Authors: Samotus O; Lee J; Jog M

Institution: London Health Sciences Centre - Lawson Health Research Institute, Department of Clinical Neurological Sciences, London, Ontario, Canada.; University of Western, Schulich School of Medicine and Dentistry, London, Ontario, Canada.

Journal: PLoS One. 2017 Jun 6;12(6):e0178670. doi: 10.1371/journal.pone.0178670. eCollection 2017.

Abstract Link: http://www.medifocus.com/abstracts.php?gid=NR013&ID=28586370

Go to http://www.medifocus.com/links/NR013/0718 for direct online access to the above Abstract Links.

130.

Assessment of Safety and Efficacy of Safinamide as a Levodopa Adjunct in Patients With Parkinson Disease and Motor Fluctuations: A Randomized Clinical Trial.

Authors:	Schapira AH; Fox SH; Hauser RA; Jankovic J; Jost WH; Kenney C; Kulisevsky J; Pahwa R; Poewe W; Anand R
Institution:	Department of Clinical Neurosciences, University College London Institute of Neurology, London, United Kingdom. University of Toronto, Toronto, Ontario, Canada. Universitat Oberta de Catalunya, Barcelona, Spain.
Journal:	JAMA Neurol. 2017 Feb 1;74(2):216-224. doi: 10.1001/jamaneurol.2016.4467.
Abstract Link:	http://www.medifocus.com/abstracts.php?gid=NR013&ID=27942720

131.

Which patients discontinue? Issues on Levodopa/carbidopa intestinal gel treatment: Italian multicentre survey of 905 patients with long-term follow-up.

Authors:	Sensi M; Cossu G; Mancini F; Pilleri M; Zibetti M; Modugno N; Quatrale R; Tamma F; Antonini A
Institution:	Department of Neurology, Azienda Ospedaliera Universitaria Arcispedale S.Anna, Ferrara, Italy. giovannicossu@aob.it. Arcugnano, Vicenza, Italy. Turin, Italy.
Journal:	Parkinsonism Relat Disord. 2017 May;38:90-92. doi: 10.1016/j.parkreldis.2017.02.020. Epub 2017 Feb 21.
Abstract Link:	http://www.medifocus.com/abstracts.php?gid=NR013&ID=28238650

132.

Dancing for Parkinson Disease: A Randomized Trial of Irish Set Dancing Compared With Usual Care.

Authors: Shanahan J; Morris ME; Bhriain ON; Volpe D; Lynch T; Clifford AM

Institution: Department of Clinical Therapies, Faculty of Education and Health Sciences, University of Limerick, Limerick, Ireland. Electronic address: joanne.s@outlook.com. and Exercise Medicine Research, School Allied Health, Melbourne, VIC, Australia. Sciences, University of Limerick, Limerick, Ireland. Ireland. University of Limerick, Limerick, Ireland.

Journal: Arch Phys Med Rehabil. 2017 Sep;98(9):1744-1751. doi: 10.1016/j.apmr.2017.02.017. Epub 2017 Mar 21.

Abstract Link: http://www.medifocus.com/abstracts.php?gid=NR013&ID=28336345

133.

Randomized trial of preladenant, given as monotherapy, in patients with early Parkinson disease.

Authors: Stocchi F; Rascol O; Hauser RA; Huyck S; Tzontcheva A; Capece R; Ho TW; Sklar P; Lines C; Michelson D; Hewitt DJ

Institution: From the Institute of Neurology (F.S.), IRCCS San Raffaele, Rome, Italy; Departments of Clinical Pharmacology and Neurosciences (O.R.), Clinical Investigation Center CIC1436, NS-Park Clinical Research Network, NeuroToul Centre of Excellence in Neurodegeneration, INSERM, Toulouse University Hospital and Toulouse University, France; Parkinson's Disease and Movement Disorders Center (R.A.H.), USF Health-Byrd Institute, Tampa, FL; and Merck & Co., Inc. (S.H., A.T., R.C., T.W.H., P.S., C.L., D.M., D.J.H.), Kenilworth, NJ. fabrizio.stocchi@fastwebnet.it.

Journal: Neurology. 2017 Jun 6;88(23):2198-2206. doi: 10.1212/WNL.0000000000004003. Epub 2017 May 10.

Abstract Link: http://www.medifocus.com/abstracts.php?gid=NR013&ID=28490648

Go to http://www.medifocus.com/links/NR013/0718 for direct online access to the above Abstract Links.

134.

Conversion to carbidopa and levodopa extended-release (IPX066) followed by its extended use in patients previously taking controlled-release carbidopa-levodopa for advanced Parkinson's disease.

Authors: Tetrud J; Nausieda P; Kreitzman D; Liang GS; Nieves A; Duker AP; Hauser RA; Farbman ES; Ellenbogen A; Hsu A; Kell S; Khanna S; Rubens R; Gupta S

Institution: The Parkinson's Institute and Clinical Center, 675 Almanor Ave, Sunnyvale, CA 94085, USA. Electronic address: jtetrud@stanford.edu.; Wisconsin Institute for Neurologic and Sleep Disorders, 945 N 12th St, Milwaukee, WI 53233, USA. Electronic address: nausiedamd@parkcent.com.; The Parkinson's Disease and Movement Disorders Center of Long Island, 283 Commack Rd, Commack, NY 11725, USA. Electronic address: PDMDCLI@aol.com.; The Parkinson's Institute and Clinical Center, 675 Almanor Ave, Sunnyvale, CA 94085, USA. Electronic address: graceliangmd@gmail.com.; Munroe Regional Medical Center, 13940 US-441, Lady Lake, FL 32159, USA. Electronic address: Anette_Nieves@munroeregional.com.

Journal: J Neurol Sci. 2017 Feb 15;373:116-123. doi: 10.1016/j.jns.2016.11.047. Epub 2016 Nov 23.

Abstract Link: http://www.medifocus.com/abstracts.php?gid=NR013&ID=28131167

135.

Timed Light Therapy for Sleep and Daytime Sleepiness Associated With Parkinson Disease: A Randomized Clinical Trial.

Authors: Videnovic A; Klerman EB; Wang W; Marconi A; Kuhta T; Zee PC

Institution: Department of Neurology, Massachusetts General Hospital, Boston 2Division of Sleep Medicine, Harvard Medical School, Boston, Massachusetts. Massachusetts3Department of Medicine, Brigham and Women's Hospital, Boston, Massachusetts.

Journal: JAMA Neurol. 2017 Apr 1;74(4):411-418. doi: 10.1001/jamaneurol.2016.5192.

Abstract Link: http://www.medifocus.com/abstracts.php?gid=NR013&ID=28241159

Go to http://www.medifocus.com/links/NR013/0718 for direct online access to the above Abstract Links.

136.

Evaluation of rotigotine transdermal patch for the treatment of apathy and motor symptoms in Parkinson's disease.

Authors: Hauser RA; Slawek J; Barone P; Dohin E; Surmann E; Asgharnejad M; Bauer L

Institution: Parkinson's Disease and Movement Disorders Center, USF Health - Byrd Institute, National Parkinson Foundation Center of Excellence, Tampa, FL, USA. rhauser@health.usf.edu. Department of Neurology, St Adalbert Hospital, Gdansk, Poland.

Journal: BMC Neurol. 2016 Jun 7;16:90. doi: 10.1186/s12883-016-0610-7.

Abstract Link: http://www.medifocus.com/abstracts.php?gid=NR013&ID=27267880

137.

Effects of rotigotine transdermal patch in patients with Parkinson's disease presenting with non-motor symptoms - results of a double-blind, randomized, placebo-controlled trial.

Authors: Antonini A; Bauer L; Dohin E; Oertel WH; Rascol O; Reichmann H; Schmid M; Singh P; Tolosa E; Chaudhuri KR

Institution: Parkinson and Movement Disorders Unit, IRCCS Hospital San Camillo, Venice, Italy. and Neurosciences, INSERM and Toulouse University Hospital, Toulouse, France. IDIBAPS, Centro de Investigacion Biomedica en Red sobre Enfermedades Neurodegenerativas (CIBERNED), Barcelona Catalonia, Spain. Hospital, Kings College and Kings Health Partners, London, UK.

Journal: Eur J Neurol. 2015 Oct;22(10):1400-7. doi: 10.1111/ene.12757. Epub 2015 Jun 22.

Abstract Link: http://www.medifocus.com/abstracts.php?gid=NR013&ID=26095948

Go to http://www.medifocus.com/links/NR013/0718 for direct online access to the above Abstract Links.

138.

Exercise for falls prevention in Parkinson disease: a randomized controlled trial.

Authors: Canning CG; Sherrington C; Lord SR; Close JC; Heritier S; Heller GZ; Howard K; Allen NE; Latt MD; Murray SM; O'Rourke SD; Paul SS; Song J; Fung VS

Institution: From the Clinical and Rehabilitation Sciences Research Group, Faculty of Health Sciences (C.G.C., N.E.A., S.M.M., S.D.O., J.S.), The George Institute for Global Health, Sydney Medical School (C.S., S.S.P.), Sydney School of Public Health (K.H.), and Sydney Medical School (S.H., V.S.C.F.), The University of Sydney, Australia; Neuroscience Research Australia and University of New South Wales (S.R.L.), Sydney; Prince of Wales Clinical School, University of New South Wales, and Neuroscience Research Australia (J.C.T.C.), Sydney; Department of Epidemiology and Preventive Medicine (S.H.), Monash University, Melbourne; Department of Statistics (G.Z.H.), Macquarie University, and Statistics Division, The George Institute for Global Health, Sydney; Department of Aged Care (M.D.L.), Royal Prince Alfred Hospital, Sydney; and Movement Disorders Unit (V.S.C.F.), Department of Neurology, Westmead Hospital, Sydney, Australia. colleen.canning@sydney.edu.au.

Journal: Neurology. 2015 Jan 20;84(3):304-12. doi: 10.1212/WNL.0000000000001155. Epub 2014 Dec 31.

Abstract Link: http://www.medifocus.com/abstracts.php?gid=NR013&ID=25552576

Go to http://www.medifocus.com/links/NR013/0718 for direct online access to the above Abstract Links.

139.

Preladenant as an Adjunctive Therapy With Levodopa in Parkinson Disease: Two Randomized Clinical Trials and Lessons Learned.

Authors: Hauser RA; Stocchi F; Rascol O; Huyck SB; Capece R; Ho TW; Sklar P; Lines C; Michelson D; Hewitt D

Institution: Parkinson's Disease and Movement Disorders Center, University of South Florida, National Parkinson Foundation Center of Excellence, Tampa. Raffaele, Rome, Italy. Medicale, Toulouse University, Toulouse, France.

Journal: JAMA Neurol. 2015 Dec;72(12):1491-500. doi: 10.1001/jamaneurol.2015.2268.

Abstract Link: http://www.medifocus.com/abstracts.php?gid=NR013&ID=26523919

140.

Economic Evaluation of a Tai Ji Quan Intervention to Reduce Falls in People With Parkinson Disease, Oregon, 2008-2011.

Authors: Li F; Harmer P

Institution: Oregon Research Institute, 1776 Millrace Dr, Eugene, OR 97403. Email: fuzhongl@ori.org.

Journal: Prev Chronic Dis. 2015 Jul 30;12:E120. doi: 10.5888/pcd12.140413.

Abstract Link: http://www.medifocus.com/abstracts.php?gid=NR013&ID=26226067

141.

Parkinson disease and risk of acute myocardial infarction: A population-based, propensity score-matched, longitudinal follow-up study.

Authors: Liang HW; Huang YP; Pan SL
Institution: Department of Physical Medicine and Rehabilitation, National Taiwan University Hospital, Taipei, Taiwan; Department of Physical Medicine and Rehabilitation, National Taiwan University College of Medicine, Taipei, Taiwan. Electronic address: panslcb@gmail.com.; Department of Physical Medicine and Rehabilitation, National Taiwan University Hospital, Yun-Lin Branch, Yunlin, Taiwan.
Journal: Am Heart J. 2015 Apr;169(4):508-14. doi: 10.1016/j.ahj.2014.11.018. Epub 2014 Dec 20.
Abstract Link: http://www.medifocus.com/abstracts.php?gid=NR013&ID=25819857

142.

Safety and tolerability of intracerebroventricular PDGF-BB in Parkinson's disease patients.

Authors: Paul G; Zachrisson O; Varrone A; Almqvist P; Jerling M; Lind G; Rehncrona S; Linderoth B; Bjartmarz H; Shafer LL; Coffey R; Svensson M; Mercer KJ; Forsberg A; Halldin C; Svenningsson P; Widner H; Frisen J; Palhagen S; Haegerstrand A
Journal: J Clin Invest. 2015 Mar 2;125(3):1339-46. doi: 10.1172/JCI79635. Epub 2015 Feb 17.
Abstract Link: http://www.medifocus.com/abstracts.php?gid=NR013&ID=25689258

Go to http://www.medifocus.com/links/NR013/0718 for direct online access to the above Abstract Links.

143.

Combined rasagiline and antidepressant use in Parkinson disease in the ADAGIO study: effects on nonmotor symptoms and tolerability.

Authors: Smith KM; Eyal E; Weintraub D
Institution: Department of Neurology, Perelman School of Medicine at the University of Pennsylvania, Philadelphia. Pennsylvania, Philadelphia3Department of Psychiatry, Perelman School of Medicine at the University of Pennsylvania, Philadelphia4Department of Veterans Affairs, Philadelphia VA Medi.
Journal: JAMA Neurol. 2015 Jan;72(1):88-95. doi: 10.1001/jamaneurol.2014.2472.
Abstract Link: http://www.medifocus.com/abstracts.php?gid=NR013&ID=25420207

144.

Feldenkrais method-based exercise improves quality of life in individuals with Parkinson's disease: a controlled, randomized clinical trial.

Authors: Teixeira-Machado L; Araujo FM; Cunha FA; Menezes M; Menezes T; Melo DeSantana J
Journal: Altern Ther Health Med. 2015 Jan-Feb;21(1):8-14.
Abstract Link: http://www.medifocus.com/abstracts.php?gid=NR013&ID=25599428

Go to http://www.medifocus.com/links/NR013/0718 for direct online access to the above Abstract Links.

145.

Prolonged-release oxycodone-naloxone for treatment of severe pain in patients with Parkinson's disease (PANDA): a double-blind, randomised, placebo-controlled trial.

Authors: Trenkwalder C; Chaudhuri KR; Martinez-Martin P; Rascol O; Ehret R; Valis M; Satori M; Krygowska-Wajs A; Marti MJ; Reimer K; Oksche A; Lomax M; DeCesare J; Hopp M

Institution: Paracelsus-Elena Hospital, Kassel, Germany; Department of Neurosurgery, University Medical Centre, Goettingen, Germany. Electronic address: ctrenkwalder@gmx.de. Hospital, London, UK; Biomedical Research Unit for Dementia, King's College, London, UK. Hospital, Toulouse, France. Faculty of Medicine in Hradec Kralove and University Hospital Hradec Kralove, Hradec Kralove, Czech Republic. Hospital Clinic, CIBERNED, Barcelona, Spain. Witten/Herdecke, Faculty of Health, Witten, Germany. Pharmacology, Justus-Liebig-Universitat Giessen, Germany.

Journal: Lancet Neurol. 2015 Dec;14(12):1161-70. doi: 10.1016/S1474-4422(15)00243-4. Epub 2015 Oct 19.

Abstract Link: http://www.medifocus.com/abstracts.php?gid=NR013&ID=26494524

146.

Low-frequency versus high-frequency subthalamic nucleus deep brain stimulation on postural control and gait in Parkinson's disease: a quantitative study.

Authors: Vallabhajosula S; Haq IU; Hwynn N; Oyama G; Okun M; Tillman MD; Hass CJ

Institution: Department of Physical Therapy Education, Elon University, Elon, NC, USA. Electronic address: svallabhajosula@elon.edu. University of Florida, Gainesville, FL, USA. Gainesville, FL, USA.

Journal: Brain Stimul. 2015 Jan-Feb;8(1):64-75. doi: 10.1016/j.brs.2014.10.011. Epub 2014 Oct 28.

Abstract Link: http://www.medifocus.com/abstracts.php?gid=NR013&ID=25440578

Go to http://www.medifocus.com/links/NR013/0718 for direct online access to the above Abstract Links.

147.

Effects of Tai Chi and Multimodal Exercise Training on Movement and Balance Function in Mild to Moderate Idiopathic Parkinson Disease.

Authors: Zhang TY; Hu Y; Nie ZY; Jin RX; Chen F; Guan Q; Hu B; Gu CY; Zhu L; Jin LJ

Institution: From the Departments of Neurology (T-YZ, YH, Z-YN, FC, QG, LZ, L-JJ) and Spine Surgery (R-XJ, BH, C-YG), Shanghai Tongji Hospital, Tongji University School of Medicine, Shanghai, China.

Journal: Am J Phys Med Rehabil. 2015 Oct;94(10 Suppl 1):921-9. doi: 10.1097/PHM.0000000000000351.

Abstract Link: http://www.medifocus.com/abstracts.php?gid=NR013&ID=26135376

Go to http://www.medifocus.com/links/NR013/0718 for direct online access to the above Abstract Links.

Deep Brain Stimulation Articles

148.

Bilateral subthalamic deep brain stimulation initial impact on nonmotor and motor symptoms in Parkinson's disease: An open prospective single institution study.

Authors: Kurcova S; Bardon J; Vastik M; Vecerkova M; Frolova M; Hvizdosova L; Nevrly M; Mensikova K; Otruba P; Krahulik D; Kurca E; Sivak S; Zapletalova J; Kanovsky P

Institution: Department of Neurology. Dentistry, Palacky University Olomouc, Czech Republic. in Bratislava and University Hospital in Martin, Slovak Republic. in Bratislava and University Hospital in Martin, Slovak Republic. University Olomouc, Czech Republic.

Journal: Medicine (Baltimore). 2018 Feb;97(5):e9750. doi: 10.1097/MD.0000000000009750.

Abstract Link: http://www.medifocus.com/abstracts.php?gid=NR013&ID=29384860

149.

Sleep-wake functions and quality of life in patients with subthalamic deep brain stimulation for Parkinson's disease.

Authors: Bargiotas P; Eugster L; Oberholzer M; Debove I; Lachenmayer ML; Mathis J; Pollo C; Schupbach WMM; Bassetti CL

Institution: Department of Neurology, University Hospital (Inselspital) and University of Bern, Bern, Switzerland.; Department of Neurosurgery, University Hospital (Inselspital) and University of Bern, Bern, Switzerland.

Journal: PLoS One. 2017 Dec 18;12(12):e0190027. doi: 10.1371/journal.pone.0190027. eCollection 2017.

Abstract Link: http://www.medifocus.com/abstracts.php?gid=NR013&ID=29253029

Go to http://www.medifocus.com/links/NR013/0718 for direct online access to the above Abstract Links.

150.

Clinical outcomes of asleep vs awake deep brain stimulation for Parkinson disease.

Authors: Brodsky MA; Anderson S; Murchison C; Seier M; Wilhelm J; Vederman A; Burchiel KJ

Institution: From the Departments of Neurology (M.A.B., S.A., C.M., M.S., J.W.) and Neurosurgery (A.V., K.J.B.), Oregon Health & Science University, Portland. brodskym@ohsu.edu.

Journal: Neurology. 2017 Nov 7;89(19):1944-1950. doi: 10.1212/WNL.0000000000004630. Epub 2017 Oct 6.

Abstract Link: http://www.medifocus.com/abstracts.php?gid=NR013&ID=28986415

151.

Parkinsonian gait improves with bilateral subthalamic nucleus deep brain stimulation during cognitive multi-tasking.

Authors: Chenji G; Wright ML; Chou KL; Seidler RD; Patil PG

Institution: Surgical Therapies Improving Movement Program, University of Michigan, Ann Arbor, MI, USA; Department of Neurosurgery, University of Michigan, Ann Arbor, MI, USA. MI, USA; School of Kinesiology, University of Michigan, Ann Arbor, MI, USA. MI, USA; Department of Neurology, University of Michigan, Ann Arbor, MI, USA; Department of Neurosurgery, University of Michigan, Ann Arbor, MI, USA. Kinesiology, University of Michigan, Ann Arbor, MI, USA. MI, USA; Department of Neurology, University of Michigan, Ann Arbor, MI, USA; Department of Neurosurgery, University of Michigan, Ann Arbor, MI, USA. Electronic address: pgpatil@med.umich.edu.

Journal: Parkinsonism Relat Disord. 2017 May;38:72-79. doi: 10.1016/j.parkreldis.2017.02.028. Epub 2017 Feb 24.

Abstract Link: http://www.medifocus.com/abstracts.php?gid=NR013&ID=28258925

152.

Key clinical milestones 15 years and onwards after DBS-STN surgery-A retrospective analysis of patients that underwent surgery between 1993 and 2001.

Authors: Constantinescu R; Eriksson B; Jansson Y; Johnels B; Holmberg B; Gudmundsdottir T; Renck A; Berglund P; Bergquist F

Institution: Department of Neurology, Institute of Neuroscience and Physiology at Sahlgrenska Academy, University of Gothenburg, Sahlgrenska University Hospital, 413 45 Goteborg, Sweden. Electronic address: Radu.Constantinescu@vgregion.se.; Department of Neurology, Norra Alvsborgs Lanssjukhus, Sjukhuskansliet, 461 85 Trollhattan, Sweden.; Department of Neuropsychiatry, Minnesmottagningen, Wallinsgatan 6, 431 41 Molndal, Sweden.

Journal: Clin Neurol Neurosurg. 2017 Mar;154:43-48. doi: 10.1016/j.clineuro.2017.01.010. Epub 2017 Jan 18.

Abstract Link: http://www.medifocus.com/abstracts.php?gid=NR013&ID=28113102

Go to http://www.medifocus.com/links/NR013/0718 for direct online access to the above Abstract Links.

153.

Thalamic deep brain stimulation for tremor in Parkinson disease, essential tremor, and dystonia.

Authors: Cury RG; Fraix V; Castrioto A; Perez Fernandez MA; Krack P; Chabardes S; Seigneuret E; Alho EJL; Benabid AL; Moro E

Institution: From the Service de Neurologie (R.G.C., V.F., A.C., M.A.P.F., E.M.), Service de Neurochirurgie (M.A.P.F., E.S.), Centre Hospitalier Universitaire de Grenoble, Universite Grenoble Alpes, INSERM U1216, Grenoble, France; Department of Neurology (R.G.C., M.A.P.F., E.J.L.A.), School of Medicine, University of Sao Paulo, Sao Paulo, Brazil; Hospital Dr. Dario Contreras (M.A.P.F.), Santo Domingo, Republica Dominicana; Service de Neurologie (P.K., S.C.), CHU de Geneve, Switzerland; and Clinatec (A.-L.B.), Centre Hospitalier Universitaire de Grenoble, France. elenamfmoro@gmail.com.

Journal: Neurology. 2017 Sep 26;89(13):1416-1423. doi: 10.1212/WNL.0000000000004295. Epub 2017 Aug 2.

Abstract Link: http://www.medifocus.com/abstracts.php?gid=NR013&ID=28768840

154.

Impulse control behaviors and subthalamic deep brain stimulation in Parkinson disease.

Authors: Merola A; Romagnolo A; Rizzi L; Rizzone MG; Zibetti M; Lanotte M; Mandybur G; Duker AP; Espay AJ; Lopiano L

Institution: Department of Neurology, Gardner Family Center for Parkinson's Disease and Movement Disorders, University of Cincinnati (UC), 260 Stetson Street, Suite 4244, Cincinnati, OH, 45219, USA. merolaae@ucmail.uc.edu.; Department of Neuroscience 'Rita Levi Montalcini', University of Turin, via Cherasco 15, 10124, Turin, Italy.; Department of Neurosurgery, Neuroscience Institute and UC College of Medicine, University of Cincinnati (UC), Cincinnati, OH, USA.

Journal: J Neurol. 2017 Jan;264(1):40-48. doi: 10.1007/s00415-016-8314-x. Epub 2016 Oct 19.

Abstract Link: http://www.medifocus.com/abstracts.php?gid=NR013&ID=27761641

Go to http://www.medifocus.com/links/NR013/0718 for direct online access to the above Abstract Links.

155.

Exploring risk factors for stuttering development in Parkinson disease after deep brain stimulation.

Authors: Picillo M; Vincos GB; Sammartino F; Lozano AM; Fasano A

Institution: Centre for Neurodegenerative Diseases (CEMAND), Department of Medicine and Surgery, Neuroscience Section, University of Salerno, Salerno, Italy. Universidad la Sabana, Bogota, Colombia. Toronto Western Hospital, University of Toronto, Canada. Toronto Western Hospital, University of Toronto, Canada; Krembil Research Institute, Toronto, Ontario, Canada. Movement Disorders Clinic, Toronto Western Hospital and Division of Neurology, University of Toronto, Toronto, Ontario, Canada; Edmond J. Safra Program in Parkinson's Disease, Toronto Western Hospital and Division of Neurology, University of Toronto, Toronto, Ontario, Canada. Electronic address: alfonso.fasano@gmail.com.

Journal: Parkinsonism Relat Disord. 2017 May;38:85-89. doi: 10.1016/j.parkreldis.2017.02.015. Epub 2017 Feb 20.

Abstract Link: http://www.medifocus.com/abstracts.php?gid=NR013&ID=28237852

156.

Apathy in patients with Parkinson's disease following deep brain stimulation of the subthalamic nucleus.

Authors: Hindle Fisher I; Pall HS; Mitchell RD; Kausar J; Cavanna AE

Institution: 1University of Birmingham Medical School,Birmingham,UK. Birmingham,Birmingham,UK. Birmingham,Birmingham,UK.

Journal: CNS Spectr. 2016 Jun;21(3):258-64. doi: 10.1017/S1092852916000171. Epub 2016 May 6.

Abstract Link: http://www.medifocus.com/abstracts.php?gid=NR013&ID=27151388

Go to http://www.medifocus.com/links/NR013/0718 for direct online access to the above Abstract Links.

157.

No Effect of Subthalamic Deep Brain Stimulation on Intertemporal Decision-Making in Parkinson Patients.

Authors: Seinstra M; Wojtecki L; Storzer L; Schnitzler A; Kalenscher T
Institution: Comparative Psychology, Institute of Experimental Psychology, Heinrich-Heine University Dusseldorf , 40225 Dusseldorf, Germany.; Institute of Clinical Neuroscience and Medical Psychology, Medical Faculty, Heinrich-Heine University Dusseldorf , 40225 Dusseldorf, Germany.
Journal: eNeuro. 2016 May 23;3(2). pii: ENEURO.0019-16.2016. doi: 10.1523/ENEURO.0019-16.2016. eCollection 2016 Mar-Apr.
Abstract Link: http://www.medifocus.com/abstracts.php?gid=NR013&ID=27257622

158.

Pallidal Deep Brain Stimulation Improves Higher Control of the Oculomotor System in Parkinson's Disease.

Authors: Antoniades CA; Rebelo P; Kennard C; Aziz TZ; Green AL; FitzGerald JJ
Institution: Nuffield Department of Clinical Neurosciences and chrystalina.antoniades@ndcn.ox.ac.uk james.fitzgerald@nds.ox.ac.uk. United Kingdom. Sciences, University of Oxford, Oxford OX3 9DU, United Kingdom. Sciences, University of Oxford, Oxford OX3 9DU, United Kingdom. Sciences, University of Oxford, Oxford OX3 9DU, United Kingdom chrystalina.antoniades@ndcn.ox.ac.uk james.fitzgerald@nds.ox.ac.uk.
Journal: J Neurosci. 2015 Sep 23;35(38):13043-52. doi: 10.1523/JNEUROSCI.2317-15.2015.
Abstract Link: http://www.medifocus.com/abstracts.php?gid=NR013&ID=26400935

Go to http://www.medifocus.com/links/NR013/0718 for direct online access to the above Abstract Links.

159.

One-year Outcome of Bilateral Subthalamic Stimulation in Parkinson Disease: An Eastern Experience.

Authors: Chiou SM; Lin YC; Huang HM
Institution: Department of Neurosurgery, China Medical University Hospital, China Medical University, Taichung, Taiwan. Electronic address: tsmchiou@pchome.com.tw. University, Taichung, Taiwan. University, Taichung, Taiwan.
Journal: World Neurosurg. 2015 Nov;84(5):1294-8. doi: 10.1016/j.wneu.2015.06.002. Epub 2015 Jun 10.
Abstract Link: http://www.medifocus.com/abstracts.php?gid=NR013&ID=26072454

160.

The long-term development of non-motor problems after STN-DBS.

Authors: Lilleeng B; Gjerstad M; Baardsen R; Dalen I; Larsen JP
Institution: The Norwegian Centre for Movement Disorders, Stavanger University Hospital, Stavanger, Norway. Stavanger, Norway. Stavanger, Norway. Stavanger, Norway. Stavanger, Norway.
Journal: Acta Neurol Scand. 2015 Oct;132(4):251-8. doi: 10.1111/ane.12391. Epub 2015 Mar 6.
Abstract Link: http://www.medifocus.com/abstracts.php?gid=NR013&ID=25752590

NOTES

Use this page for taking notes as you review your Guidebook

4 - Centers of Research

This section of your *MediFocus Guidebook* is a unique directory of doctors, researchers, medical centers, and research institutions with specialized research interest, and in many cases, clinical expertise in the management of this specific medical condition. The *Centers of Research* directory is a valuable resource for quickly identifying and locating leading medical authorities and medical institutions within the United States and other countries that are considered to be at the forefront in clinical research and treatment of this disorder.

Use the *Centers of Research* directory to contact, consult, or network with leading experts in the field and to locate a hospital or medical center that can help you.

The following information is provided in the *Centers of Research* directory:

- **Geographic Location**
    - United States: the information is divided by individual states listed in alphabetical order. Not all states may be included.
    - Other Countries: information is presented for select countries worldwide listed in alphabetical order. Not all countries may be included.

- **Names of Authors**
    - Select names of individual authors (doctors, researchers, or other health-care professionals) with specialized research interest, and in many cases, clinical expertise in the management of this specific medical condition, who have recently published articles in leading medical journals about the condition.
    - E-mail addresses for individual authors, if listed on their specific publications, is also provided.

- **Institutional Affiliations**
    - Next to each individual author's name is their **institutional affiliation** (hospital, medical center, or research institution) where the study was conducted as listed in their publication(s).

- In many cases, information about the specific **department** within the medical institution where the individual author was located at the time the study was conducted is also provided.

Centers of Research

United States

AZ - Arizona

Name of Author	Institutional Affiliation
Troster AI	Department of Clinical Neuropsychology and Center for Neuromodulation, Barrow Neurological Institute, Phoenix, AZ, USA.

FL - Florida

Name of Author	Institutional Affiliation
Borlongan CV	a Center of Excellence for Aging and Brain Repair, Department of Neurosurgery and Brain Repair, University of South Florida College of Medicine, Tampa, FL, USA.
Getz SJ	Department of Neurology, Division of Neuropsychology, University of Miami Miller School of Medicine, Miami, FL, USA. School of Medicine, Miami, FL, USA.
Grundmann O	a Department of Medicinal Chemistry , College of Pharmacy, University of Florida , Gainesville , FL , USA. , Gainesville , FL , USA.
Gupta S	The Parkinson's Institute and Clinical Center, 675 Almanor Ave, Sunnyvale, CA 94085, USA. Electronic address: jtetrud@stanford.edu.; Wisconsin Institute for Neurologic and Sleep Disorders, 945 N 12th St, Milwaukee, WI 53233, USA. Electronic address: nausiedamd@parkcent.com.; The Parkinson's Disease and Movement Disorders Center of Long Island, 283 Commack Rd, Commack, NY 11725, USA. Electronic address: PDMDCLI@aol.com.; The Parkinson's Institute and Clinical Center, 675 Almanor Ave, Sunnyvale, CA 94085, USA. Electronic address: graceliangmd@gmail.com.; Munroe Regional Medical Center, 13940 US-441, Lady Lake, FL 32159, USA. Electronic address: Anette_Nieves@munroeregional.com.

Name of Author	Institutional Affiliation
Hass CJ	Department of Physical Therapy Education, Elon University, Elon, NC, USA. Electronic address: svallabhajosula@elon.edu. University of Florida, Gainesville, FL, USA. Gainesville, FL, USA.
Levin B	Department of Neurology, Division of Neuropsychology, University of Miami Miller School of Medicine, Miami, FL, USA. School of Medicine, Miami, FL, USA.
Morgan LA	a Department of Medicinal Chemistry , College of Pharmacy, University of Florida , Gainesville , FL , USA. , Gainesville , FL , USA.
Pantcheva P	a Center of Excellence for Aging and Brain Repair, Department of Neurosurgery and Brain Repair, University of South Florida College of Medicine, Tampa, FL, USA.
Tetrud J	The Parkinson's Institute and Clinical Center, 675 Almanor Ave, Sunnyvale, CA 94085, USA. Electronic address: jtetrud@stanford.edu.; Wisconsin Institute for Neurologic and Sleep Disorders, 945 N 12th St, Milwaukee, WI 53233, USA. Electronic address: nausiedamd@parkcent.com.; The Parkinson's Disease and Movement Disorders Center of Long Island, 283 Commack Rd, Commack, NY 11725, USA. Electronic address: PDMDCLI@aol.com.; The Parkinson's Institute and Clinical Center, 675 Almanor Ave, Sunnyvale, CA 94085, USA. Electronic address: graceliangmd@gmail.com.; Munroe Regional Medical Center, 13940 US-441, Lady Lake, FL 32159, USA. Electronic address: Anette_Nieves@munroeregional.com.
Vallabhajosula S	Department of Physical Therapy Education, Elon University, Elon, NC, USA. Electronic address: svallabhajosula@elon.edu. University of Florida, Gainesville, FL, USA. Gainesville, FL, USA.

IA - Iowa

Name of Author	Institutional Affiliation
Stegemoller EL	Iowa State University.
Williams EK	Iowa State University.

IL - Illinois

Name of Author	Institutional Affiliation
Herring WJ	*Merck & Co, Inc, Kenilworth, NJ; daggerQUEST Research Institute, Bingham Farms, MI; and double daggerRush University Medical Center, Chicago, IL.
Kianirad Y	Department of Neurology, Feinberg School of Medicine, Northwestern University, Chicago, IL, USA. Yasaman.Kianirad@northwestern.edu. Feinberg School of Medicine, Northwestern University, Abbott Hall 11th Floor, 710 North Lake Shore Drive, Chicago, IL, 60611, USA. TSimuni@nm.org.
Simuni T	Department of Neurology, Feinberg School of Medicine, Northwestern University, Chicago, IL, USA. Yasaman.Kianirad@northwestern.edu. Feinberg School of Medicine, Northwestern University, Abbott Hall 11th Floor, 710 North Lake Shore Drive, Chicago, IL, 60611, USA. TSimuni@nm.org.
Verhagen Metman L	*Merck & Co, Inc, Kenilworth, NJ; daggerQUEST Research Institute, Bingham Farms, MI; and double daggerRush University Medical Center, Chicago, IL.

MA - Massachussetts

Name of Author	Institutional Affiliation
Ellis JM	Department of Discovery Chemistry, Merck & Co., Inc., 33 Avenue Louis Pasteur, Boston, MA 02115, USA. Electronic address: michael_ellis@merck.com. Boston, MA 02115, USA.
Fell MJ	Department of Discovery Chemistry, Merck & Co., Inc., 33 Avenue Louis Pasteur, Boston, MA 02115, USA. Electronic address: michael_ellis@merck.com. Boston, MA 02115, USA.
Sahli ZT	a Department of Psychiatry and Neuroscience Program , Harvard Medical School, McLean Hospital , Belmont , MA , USA. McLean Hospital , Belmont , MA , USA.
Tarazi FI	a Department of Psychiatry and Neuroscience Program , Harvard Medical School, McLean Hospital , Belmont , MA , USA. McLean Hospital , Belmont , MA , USA.
Videnovic A	Department of Neurology, Massachusetts General Hospital, Boston 2Division of Sleep Medicine, Harvard Medical School, Boston, Massachusetts. Massachusetts3Department of Medicine, Brigham and Women's Hospital, Boston, Massachusetts.
Zee PC	Department of Neurology, Massachusetts General Hospital, Boston 2Division of Sleep Medicine, Harvard Medical School, Boston, Massachusetts. Massachusetts3Department of Medicine, Brigham and Women's Hospital, Boston, Massachusetts.

MI - Michigan

Name of Author	Institutional Affiliation
Brundin P	Van Andel Research Institute, Translational Parkinson's Disease Research, Center for Neurodegenerative Science, 333 Bostwick Avenue NE, Grand Rapids, MI 49503, USA.

Name of Author	Institutional Affiliation
Chenji G	Surgical Therapies Improving Movement Program, University of Michigan, Ann Arbor, MI, USA; Department of Neurosurgery, University of Michigan, Ann Arbor, MI, USA. MI, USA; School of Kinesiology, University of Michigan, Ann Arbor, MI, USA. MI, USA; Department of Neurology, University of Michigan, Ann Arbor, MI, USA; Department of Neurosurgery, University of Michigan, Ann Arbor, MI, USA. Kinesiology, University of Michigan, Ann Arbor, MI, USA. MI, USA; Department of Neurology, University of Michigan, Ann Arbor, MI, USA; Department of Neurosurgery, University of Michigan, Ann Arbor, MI, USA. Electronic address: pgpatil@med.umich.edu.
Patil PG	Surgical Therapies Improving Movement Program, University of Michigan, Ann Arbor, MI, USA; Department of Neurosurgery, University of Michigan, Ann Arbor, MI, USA. MI, USA; School of Kinesiology, University of Michigan, Ann Arbor, MI, USA. MI, USA; Department of Neurology, University of Michigan, Ann Arbor, MI, USA; Department of Neurosurgery, University of Michigan, Ann Arbor, MI, USA. Kinesiology, University of Michigan, Ann Arbor, MI, USA. MI, USA; Department of Neurology, University of Michigan, Ann Arbor, MI, USA; Department of Neurosurgery, University of Michigan, Ann Arbor, MI, USA. Electronic address: pgpatil@med.umich.edu.
Silver DE	From the Coastal Neurological Medical Group, Inc. (D.E.S.), La Jolla, CA; and the Parkinson's and Movement Disorders Center (R.M.T.), Farmington Hills, MI. richardtrosch@comcast.net.
Trosch RM	From the Coastal Neurological Medical Group, Inc. (D.E.S.), La Jolla, CA; and the Parkinson's and Movement Disorders Center (R.M.T.), Farmington Hills, MI. richardtrosch@comcast.net.
Wyse R	Van Andel Research Institute, Translational Parkinson's Disease Research, Center for Neurodegenerative Science, 333 Bostwick Avenue NE, Grand Rapids, MI 49503, USA.

MN - Minnesota

Name of Author	Institutional Affiliation
Dalvin LA	Department of Ophthalmology, Mayo Clinic, Rochester, MN. Center, Rochester, MN. Jacksonville, FL. Medicine, Mayo Clinic, Rochester, MN. Electronic address: pulido.jose@mayo.edu.
Jabbari B	Department of Neurology, Mayo Clinic, Rochester, MN. Electronic address: shivamommittal@gmail.com.
Mittal SO	Department of Neurology, Mayo Clinic, Rochester, MN. Electronic address: shivamommittal@gmail.com.
Pulido JS	Department of Ophthalmology, Mayo Clinic, Rochester, MN. Center, Rochester, MN. Jacksonville, FL. Medicine, Mayo Clinic, Rochester, MN. Electronic address: pulido.jose@mayo.edu.

NE - Nebraska

Name of Author	Institutional Affiliation
Dawson JD	From the Departments of Neurology (E.Y.U., M.R., S.W.A.) and Biostatistics (A.M.J.O., J.D.D.), University of Iowa; Neurology Service (E.Y.U.) and Comprehensive Access and Delivery Research & Evaluation (A.M.J.O.), Veterans Affairs Medical Center, Iowa City, IA; and Department of Neurology (M.R.), University of Nebraska, Omaha. ergun-uc@uiowa.edu.
Uc EY	From the Departments of Neurology (E.Y.U., M.R., S.W.A.) and Biostatistics (A.M.J.O., J.D.D.), University of Iowa; Neurology Service (E.Y.U.) and Comprehensive Access and Delivery Research & Evaluation (A.M.J.O.), Veterans Affairs Medical Center, Iowa City, IA; and Department of Neurology (M.R.), University of Nebraska, Omaha. ergun-uc@uiowa.edu.

NJ - New Jersey

Name of Author	Institutional Affiliation
Hewitt DJ	From the Institute of Neurology (F.S.), IRCCS San Raffaele, Rome, Italy; Departments of Clinical Pharmacology and Neurosciences (O.R.), Clinical Investigation Center CIC1436, NS-Park Clinical Research Network, NeuroToul Centre of Excellence in Neurodegeneration, INSERM, Toulouse University Hospital and Toulouse University, France; Parkinson's Disease and Movement Disorders Center (R.A.H.), USF Health-Byrd Institute, Tampa, FL; and Merck & Co., Inc. (S.H., A.T., R.C., T.W.H., P.S., C.L., D.M., D.J.H.), Kenilworth, NJ. fabrizio.stocchi@fastwebnet.it.
Stocchi F	From the Institute of Neurology (F.S.), IRCCS San Raffaele, Rome, Italy; Departments of Clinical Pharmacology and Neurosciences (O.R.), Clinical Investigation Center CIC1436, NS-Park Clinical Research Network, NeuroToul Centre of Excellence in Neurodegeneration, INSERM, Toulouse University Hospital and Toulouse University, France; Parkinson's Disease and Movement Disorders Center (R.A.H.), USF Health-Byrd Institute, Tampa, FL; and Merck & Co., Inc. (S.H., A.T., R.C., T.W.H., P.S., C.L., D.M., D.J.H.), Kenilworth, NJ. fabrizio.stocchi@fastwebnet.it.

NY - New York

Name of Author	Institutional Affiliation
Brucker BM	Department of Urology, New York University Langone Medical Center, 150 East 32nd street second floor, New York, NY 10016, USA; Department of Obstetrics and Gynecology, New York University Langone Medical Center, 550 First Avenue, New York, NY 10016, USA. Electronic address: Benjamin.Brucker@nyumc.org. street second floor, New York, NY 10016, USA.

Name of Author	Institutional Affiliation
Dhall R	From the Parkinson's Institute and Clinical Center (R.D.), Sunnyvale, CA; and Parkinson's Disease and Movement Disorder Center of Long Island (D.L.K.), Commack, NY. drdhall@gmail.com.
DiFrancisco-Donoghue J	Department of Osteopathic Medicine, College of Osteopathic Medicine, New York Institute of Technology (NYITCOM), Old Westbury, NY, USA. Westbury, NY, USA. Westbury, NY, USA. USA. Institute of Technology (NYITCOM), Old Westbury, NY, USA. Institute of Technology (NYITCOM), Old Westbury, NY, USA.
Fahn S	From the Department of Neurology (P.A.L.), Henry Ford Hospital; Department of Neurology (P.A.L.), Wayne State University School of Medicine, Detroit, MI; and Department of Neurology (S.F.), Columbia University Medical Center, New York, NY. plewitt1@hfhs.org.
Kalra S	Department of Urology, New York University Langone Medical Center, 150 East 32nd street second floor, New York, NY 10016, USA; Department of Obstetrics and Gynecology, New York University Langone Medical Center, 550 First Avenue, New York, NY 10016, USA. Electronic address: Benjamin.Brucker@nyumc.org. street second floor, New York, NY 10016, USA.
Katz R	Clintrex LLC, United States; Dept of Neurology, Dept of Neuroscience, Mount Sinai School of Medicine, New York, NY, United States. Electronic address: Warren.olanow@mssm.edu. States. States.
Kreitzman DL	From the Parkinson's Institute and Clinical Center (R.D.), Sunnyvale, CA; and Parkinson's Disease and Movement Disorder Center of Long Island (D.L.K.), Commack, NY. drdhall@gmail.com.
LeWitt PA	From the Department of Neurology (P.A.L.), Henry Ford Hospital; Department of Neurology (P.A.L.), Wayne State University School of Medicine, Detroit, MI; and Department of Neurology (S.F.), Columbia University Medical Center, New York, NY. plewitt1@hfhs.org.

Name of Author	Institutional Affiliation
Olanow CW	Clintrex LLC, United States; Dept of Neurology, Dept of Neuroscience, Mount Sinai School of Medicine, New York, NY, United States. Electronic address: Warren.olanow@mssm.edu. States. States.
Petsko GA	Taub Institute for Research on Alzheimer's Disease and the Ageing Brain, Departments of Neurology, Radiology, and Psychiatry, Columbia University College of Physicians and Surgeons, New York, New York 10032, USA. Neurology and Feil Family Brain and Mind Research Institute, Weill Cornell Medical College, New York, New York 10065, USA.
Small SA	Taub Institute for Research on Alzheimer's Disease and the Ageing Brain, Departments of Neurology, Radiology, and Psychiatry, Columbia University College of Physicians and Surgeons, New York, New York 10032, USA. Neurology and Feil Family Brain and Mind Research Institute, Weill Cornell Medical College, New York, New York 10065, USA.
Yao S	Department of Osteopathic Medicine, College of Osteopathic Medicine, New York Institute of Technology (NYITCOM), Old Westbury, NY, USA. Westbury, NY, USA. Westbury, NY, USA. USA. Institute of Technology (NYITCOM), Old Westbury, NY, USA. Institute of Technology (NYITCOM), Old Westbury, NY, USA.

OR - Oregon

Name of Author	Institutional Affiliation
Brodsky MA	From the Departments of Neurology (M.A.B., S.A., C.M., M.S., J.W.) and Neurosurgery (A.V., K.J.B.), Oregon Health & Science University, Portland. brodskym@ohsu.edu.
Burchiel KJ	From the Departments of Neurology (M.A.B., S.A., C.M., M.S., J.W.) and Neurosurgery (A.V., K.J.B.), Oregon Health & Science University, Portland. brodskym@ohsu.edu.

Name of Author	Institutional Affiliation
Harmer P	Oregon Research Institute, 1776 Millrace Dr, Eugene, OR 97403. Email: fuzhongl@ori.org.
Li F	Oregon Research Institute, 1776 Millrace Dr, Eugene, OR 97403. Email: fuzhongl@ori.org.

PA - Pennsylvania

Name of Author	Institutional Affiliation
Smith KM	Department of Neurology, Perelman School of Medicine at the University of Pennsylvania, Philadelphia. Pennsylvania, Philadelphia3Department of Psychiatry, Perelman School of Medicine at the University of Pennsylvania, Philadelphia4Department of Veterans Affairs, Philadelphia VA Medi.
Weintraub D	Department of Neurology, Perelman School of Medicine at the University of Pennsylvania, Philadelphia. Pennsylvania, Philadelphia3Department of Psychiatry, Perelman School of Medicine at the University of Pennsylvania, Philadelphia4Department of Veterans Affairs, Philadelphia VA Medi.

RI - Rhode Island

Name of Author	Institutional Affiliation
Frakey LL	From the Memorial Hospital of Rhode Island-Medical Rehabilitation, Pawtucket, R.I. (LLF); and the Alpert Medical School of Brown University, Providence, R.I. (JHF).
Friedman JH	a Movement Disorders Program , Butler Hospital , Providence , RI , USA. Providence , RI , USA.

VA - Virginia

Name of Author	Institutional Affiliation
Bond AE	Department of Neurosurgery, University of Virginia Health Science Center, Charlottesville. Charlottesville. Charlottesville. Charlottesville. Charlottesville. Charlottesville. Charlottesville. Center, Charlottesville. Charlottesville.
Bozymski KM	1 Virginia Commonwealth University Health System/Medical College of Virginia Hospitals, Richmond, VA, USA. Hospitals, Richmond, VA, USA. Hospitals, Richmond, VA, USA. Hospitals, Richmond, VA, USA. Hospitals, Richmond, VA, USA.
Crouse EL	1 Virginia Commonwealth University Health System/Medical College of Virginia Hospitals, Richmond, VA, USA. Hospitals, Richmond, VA, USA. Hospitals, Richmond, VA, USA. Hospitals, Richmond, VA, USA. Hospitals, Richmond, VA, USA.
Elias WJ	Department of Neurosurgery, University of Virginia Health Science Center, Charlottesville. Charlottesville. Charlottesville. Charlottesville. Charlottesville. Charlottesville. Charlottesville. Center, Charlottesville. Charlottesville.

WA - Washington

Name of Author	Institutional Affiliation
Agarwal P	a College of Medical and Dental Sciences , University of Birmingham , Birmingham , UK. Kirkland , WA , USA. Kirkland , WA , USA. Kirkland , WA , USA.
Madan A	a College of Medical and Dental Sciences , University of Birmingham , Birmingham , UK. Kirkland , WA , USA. Kirkland , WA , USA. Kirkland , WA , USA.

WV - West Virginia

Name of Author	Institutional Affiliation
Miller DB	Centers for Disease Control and Prevention, National Institute for Occupational Safety and Health, Morgantown, WV 26505. Electronic address: dum6@cdc.gov. Safety and Health, Morgantown, WV 26505. Electronic address: jdo5@cdc.gov.
O'Callaghan JP	Centers for Disease Control and Prevention, National Institute for Occupational Safety and Health, Morgantown, WV 26505. Electronic address: dum6@cdc.gov. Safety and Health, Morgantown, WV 26505. Electronic address: jdo5@cdc.gov.

Centers of Research

Other Countries

Australia

Name of Author	Institutional Affiliation
Canning CG	From the Clinical and Rehabilitation Sciences Research Group, Faculty of Health Sciences (C.G.C., N.E.A., S.M.M., S.D.O., J.S.), The George Institute for Global Health, Sydney Medical School (C.S., S.S.P.), Sydney School of Public Health (K.H.), and Sydney Medical School (S.H., V.S.C.F.), The University of Sydney, Australia; Neuroscience Research Australia and University of New South Wales (S.R.L.), Sydney; Prince of Wales Clinical School, University of New South Wales, and Neuroscience Research Australia (J.C.T.C.), Sydney; Department of Epidemiology and Preventive Medicine (S.H.), Monash University, Melbourne; Department of Statistics (G.Z.H.), Macquarie University, and Statistics Division, The George Institute for Global Health, Sydney; Department of Aged Care (M.D.L.), Royal Prince Alfred Hospital, Sydney; and Movement Disorders Unit (V.S.C.F.), Department of Neurology, Westmead Hospital, Sydney, Australia. colleen.canning@sydney.edu.au.

Name of Author	Institutional Affiliation
Fung VS	From the Clinical and Rehabilitation Sciences Research Group, Faculty of Health Sciences (C.G.C., N.E.A., S.M.M., S.D.O., J.S.), The George Institute for Global Health, Sydney Medical School (C.S., S.S.P.), Sydney School of Public Health (K.H.), and Sydney Medical School (S.H., V.S.C.F.), The University of Sydney, Australia; Neuroscience Research Australia and University of New South Wales (S.R.L.), Sydney; Prince of Wales Clinical School, University of New South Wales, and Neuroscience Research Australia (J.C.T.C.), Sydney; Department of Epidemiology and Preventive Medicine (S.H.), Monash University, Melbourne; Department of Statistics (G.Z.H.), Macquarie University, and Statistics Division, The George Institute for Global Health, Sydney; Department of Aged Care (M.D.L.), Royal Prince Alfred Hospital, Sydney; and Movement Disorders Unit (V.S.C.F.), Department of Neurology, Westmead Hospital, Sydney, Australia. colleen.canning@sydney.edu.au.
Lampit A	From the Regenerative Neuroscience Group (I.H.K.L., H.H., M.V., A.L.) and Parkinson's Disease Research Clinic (C.C.W., S.J.G.L.), Brain and Mind Centre, University of Sydney, Australia. amit.lampit@sydney.edu.au.
Leung IH	From the Regenerative Neuroscience Group (I.H.K.L., H.H., M.V., A.L.) and Parkinson's Disease Research Clinic (C.C.W., S.J.G.L.), Brain and Mind Centre, University of Sydney, Australia. amit.lampit@sydney.edu.au.

Brazil

Name of Author	Institutional Affiliation
Aroxa FH	Academic of Medicine graduation of Federal University of Pernambuco - Recife, Pernambuco (PE), Brazil. Recife (PE), Brazil. Recife (PE), Brazil. Recife (PE), Brazil. Recife (PE), Brazil. Brazil. Electronic address: nadjaasano@gmail.com.
Asano NM	Academic of Medicine graduation of Federal University of Pernambuco - Recife, Pernambuco (PE), Brazil. Recife (PE), Brazil. Recife (PE), Brazil. Recife (PE), Brazil. Recife (PE), Brazil. Brazil. Electronic address: nadjaasano@gmail.com.
Bassani TB	Pontificia Universidade Catolica do Parana, Curitiba, PR, Brazil. Brazil.
Christofoletti G	From the Graduate Program in Health and Development, Universidade Federal de Mato Grosso do Sul, UFMS, Campo Grande, Mato Grosso do Sul (RTO, LAF, GC); Universidade Estadual Paulista, UNESP, Rio Claro (LTBG, FAB); and Universidade Estadual Paulista, UNESP, Bauru, Sao Paulo, Brazil (FAB).
Nassif DV	Department of Neurology, Pedro Ernesto University Hospital, State University of Rio de Janeiro, Rio de Janeiro, Brazil. Rio de Janeiro, Rio de Janeiro, Brazil.
Pereira JS	Department of Neurology, Pedro Ernesto University Hospital, State University of Rio de Janeiro, Rio de Janeiro, Brazil. Rio de Janeiro, Rio de Janeiro, Brazil.
Rauh LK	Pontificia Universidade Catolica do Parana, Curitiba, PR, Brazil. Brazil.
da Silva FC	University of State of Santa Catarina, Center for Health Sciences and Sports, Adapted Physical Activity Laboratory, Florianopolis, Santa Catarina, Brazil.; University of Brasilia, Faculty of Physical Education, Brasilia, Brazil.; University of Southern Santa Catarina, Medicine Course, Florianopolis, Santa Catarina, Brazil.

Name of Author	Institutional Affiliation
da Silva R	University of State of Santa Catarina, Center for Health Sciences and Sports, Adapted Physical Activity Laboratory, Florianopolis, Santa Catarina, Brazil.; University of Brasilia, Faculty of Physical Education, Brasilia, Brazil.; University of Southern Santa Catarina, Medicine Course, Florianopolis, Santa Catarina, Brazil.
de Oliveira RT	From the Graduate Program in Health and Development, Universidade Federal de Mato Grosso do Sul, UFMS, Campo Grande, Mato Grosso do Sul (RTO, LAF, GC); Universidade Estadual Paulista, UNESP, Rio Claro (LTBG, FAB); and Universidade Estadual Paulista, UNESP, Bauru, Sao Paulo, Brazil (FAB).

Canada

Name of Author	Institutional Affiliation
Bari AA	a 1 Division of Neurosurgery, Department of Surgery, Toronto Western Hospital, Krembil Neuroscience Center, University of Toronto, Toronto, ON M5T 2S8, Canada.; b 2 Morton and Gloria Shulman Movement Disorders Clinic and the Edmond J. Safra Program in Parkinson's Disease, Toronto Western Hospital, UHN, Division of Neurology, University of Toronto, Toronto, ON M5T 2S8, Canada.
Bognar S	a Department of Physical Therapy , University of Toronto , Toronto , Canada. , Canada.
Ensom MHH	1 Qatar University, Doha, Qatar. Canada.
Evans C	a Department of Physical Therapy , University of Toronto , Toronto , Canada. , Canada.
Farrer MJ	Department of Medical Genetics, Centre for Applied Neurogenetics, Djavad Mowafaghian Centre for Brain Health, University of British Columbia, Vancouver, BC, Canada. Electronic address: mfarrer@can.ubc.ca.; Division of Neurology, Centre for Applied Neurogenetics, Djavad Mowafaghian Centre for Brain Health, University of British Columbia, Vancouver, BC, Canada.

Name of Author	**Institutional Affiliation**
Fasano A	Centre for Neurodegenerative Diseases (CEMAND), Department of Medicine and Surgery, Neuroscience Section, University of Salerno, Salerno, Italy. Universidad la Sabana, Bogota, Colombia. Toronto Western Hospital, University of Toronto, Canada. Toronto Western Hospital, University of Toronto, Canada; Krembil Research Institute, Toronto, Ontario, Canada. Movement Disorders Clinic, Toronto Western Hospital and Division of Neurology, University of Toronto, Toronto, Ontario, Canada; Edmond J. Safra Program in Parkinson's Disease, Toronto Western Hospital and Division of Neurology, University of Toronto, Toronto, Ontario, Canada. Electronic address: alfonso.fasano@gmail.com.
Gagnon JF	Department of Psychology, Universite du Quebec a Montreal, Montreal, QC, Canada. Montreal, Montreal, QC, Canada. Montreal, Montreal, QC, Canada. de Montreal, Montreal, QC, Canada. de Montreal, Montreal, QC, Canada. Montreal, Montreal, QC, Canada. Montreal, Montreal, QC, Canada.
Honey CR	1Division of Neurosurgery,University of British Columbia,Vancouver,British Columbia. of Alberta,Edmonton,Alberta. Program in Parkinson's Disease,Toronto Western Hospital,University Health Network,Toronto,Ontario. Program in Parkinson's Disease,Toronto Western Hospital,University Health Network,Toronto,Ontario. Program in Parkinson's Disease,Toronto Western Hospital,University Health Network,Toronto,Ontario. Montreal Health Centre,Montreal,Quebec,Canada.
Jog M	London Health Sciences Centre - Lawson Health Research Institute, Department of Clinical Neurological Sciences, London, Ontario, Canada.; University of Western, Schulich School of Medicine and Dentistry, London, Ontario, Canada.

Name of Author	Institutional Affiliation
Jozwiak N	Department of Psychology, Universite du Quebec a Montreal, Montreal, QC, Canada. Montreal, Montreal, QC, Canada. Montreal, Montreal, QC, Canada. de Montreal, Montreal, QC, Canada. de Montreal, Montreal, QC, Canada. Montreal, Montreal, QC, Canada. Montreal, Montreal, QC, Canada.
Kaminska M	From Clinica Alemana de Santiago (V.P.M.), Facultad de Medicina, Universidad del Desarrollo, Santiago, Chile; and Respiratory Division & Sleep Laboratory (P.G., A.R., R.J.K., M.K.), Montreal Neurological Hospital (A.-L.L.), Departments of Medicine and Epidemiology, Biostatistics & Occupational Health (A.B.), and Respiratory Epidemiology and Clinical Research Unit, Research Institute (A.B., M.K.), McGill University Health Centre, Montreal, Canada. vmery@alemana.cl.
Lang AE	From the Department of Neurology, Montreal General Hospital (R.B.P., A.P.), and Department of Epidemiology and Biostatistics (L.J.), McGill University, Montreal; Department of Neurology (J.A., A.B., D.H.), University of Manitoba, Winnipeg, Canada; Pontifical Catholic University of Parana (M.M., A.M.), Curitiba, Brazil; Department of Neurology (D.G.), Ottawa Hospital, University of Ottawa Brain and Mind Research Institute; Department of Neurology (S.F.), University of Calgary; Division of Neurology (R.P.M., A.E.L.), Toronto Western Hospital; and Department of Medicine, Division of Neurology, Djavad Mowafaghian Centre for Brain Health, and Pacific Parkinson's Research Centre (S.A.-C.), University of British Columbia, Vancouver, Canada. ron.postuma@mcgill.ca.
Lozano AM	a 1 Division of Neurosurgery, Department of Surgery, Toronto Western Hospital, Krembil Neuroscience Center, University of Toronto, Toronto, ON M5T 2S8, Canada.; b 2 Morton and Gloria Shulman Movement Disorders Clinic and the Edmond J. Safra Program in Parkinson's Disease, Toronto Western Hospital, UHN, Division of Neurology, University of Toronto, Toronto, ON M5T 2S8, Canada.

Name of Author	Institutional Affiliation
Marras C	a Toronto Western Hospital, Morton and Gloria Shulman Movement Disorders Centre, 399 Bathurst Street, Toronto, Ontario, Canada.
Mery VP	From Clinica Alemana de Santiago (V.P.M.), Facultad de Medicina, Universidad del Desarrollo, Santiago, Chile; and Respiratory Division & Sleep Laboratory (P.G., A.R., R.J.K., M.K.), Montreal Neurological Hospital (A.-L.L.), Departments of Medicine and Epidemiology, Biostatistics & Occupational Health (A.B.), and Respiratory Epidemiology and Clinical Research Unit, Research Institute (A.B., M.K.), McGill University Health Centre, Montreal, Canada. vmery@alemana.cl.
Panisset M	1Division of Neurosurgery,University of British Columbia,Vancouver,British Columbia. of Alberta,Edmonton,Alberta. Program in Parkinson's Disease,Toronto Western Hospital,University Health Network,Toronto,Ontario. Program in Parkinson's Disease,Toronto Western Hospital,University Health Network,Toronto,Ontario. Program in Parkinson's Disease,Toronto Western Hospital,University Health Network,Toronto,Ontario. Montreal Health Centre,Montreal,Quebec,Canada.
Picillo M	Centre for Neurodegenerative Diseases (CEMAND), Department of Medicine and Surgery, Neuroscience Section, University of Salerno, Salerno, Italy. Universidad la Sabana, Bogota, Colombia. Toronto Western Hospital, University of Toronto, Canada. Toronto Western Hospital, University of Toronto, Canada; Krembil Research Institute, Toronto, Ontario, Canada. Movement Disorders Clinic, Toronto Western Hospital and Division of Neurology, University of Toronto, Toronto, Ontario, Canada; Edmond J. Safra Program in Parkinson's Disease, Toronto Western Hospital and Division of Neurology, University of Toronto, Toronto, Ontario, Canada. Electronic address: alfonso.fasano@gmail.com.

Name of Author	Institutional Affiliation
Postuma RB	From the Department of Neurology, Montreal General Hospital (R.B.P., A.P.), and Department of Epidemiology and Biostatistics (L.J.), McGill University, Montreal; Department of Neurology (J.A., A.B., D.H.), University of Manitoba, Winnipeg, Canada; Pontifical Catholic University of Parana (M.M., A.M.), Curitiba, Brazil; Department of Neurology (D.G.), Ottawa Hospital, University of Ottawa Brain and Mind Research Institute; Department of Neurology (S.F.), University of Calgary; Division of Neurology (R.P.M., A.E.L.), Toronto Western Hospital; and Department of Medicine, Division of Neurology, Djavad Mowafaghian Centre for Brain Health, and Pacific Parkinson's Research Centre (S.A.-C.), University of British Columbia, Vancouver, Canada. ron.postuma@mcgill.ca.
Samotus O	London Health Sciences Centre - Lawson Health Research Institute, Department of Clinical Neurological Sciences, London, Ontario, Canada.; University of Western, Schulich School of Medicine and Dentistry, London, Ontario, Canada.
Visanji N	a Toronto Western Hospital, Morton and Gloria Shulman Movement Disorders Centre, 399 Bathurst Street, Toronto, Ontario, Canada.
Volta M	Department of Medical Genetics, Centre for Applied Neurogenetics, Djavad Mowafaghian Centre for Brain Health, University of British Columbia, Vancouver, BC, Canada. Electronic address: mfarrer@can.ubc.ca.; Division of Neurology, Centre for Applied Neurogenetics, Djavad Mowafaghian Centre for Brain Health, University of British Columbia, Vancouver, BC, Canada.
Wilby KJ	1 Qatar University, Doha, Qatar. Canada.

China

Name of Author	Institutional Affiliation
Bai J	Department of Neurology, Hebei Province Cangzhou Hospital of Integrated Traditional and Western Medicine, Cangzhou, China.; Dongzhimen Hospital, Beijing University of Chinese Medicine, Beijing, China.
Cai J	College of Integrative Medicine, Fujian University of Traditional Chinese Medicine, Fuzhou, 350122, China. 441000, China. Province, 364000, China. Fuzhou, 350003, China. Medicine, Fuzhou, 350122, China. caij1@163.com.
Jin LJ	From the Departments of Neurology (T-YZ, YH, Z-YN, FC, QG, LZ, L-JJ) and Spine Surgery (R-XJ, BH, C-YG), Shanghai Tongji Hospital, Tongji University School of Medicine, Shanghai, China.
Li BD	Department of Neurology, Hebei Province Cangzhou Hospital of Integrated Traditional and Western Medicine, Cangzhou, China.; Dongzhimen Hospital, Beijing University of Chinese Medicine, Beijing, China.
Li D	Department of Functional Neurosurgery, Ruijin Hospital, Shanghai Jiao Tong University School of Medicine, Shanghai, China.
Li S	aDepartment of Acupuncture, China-Japan Friendship Hospital, Beijing bDepartment of Neurology, The Affiliated Hospital of Yangzhou University, Yangzhou University, Yangzhou, Jiangsu Province cDepartment of Orthopedics, Tumd Right Banner Hospital, Baotou City dDepartment of Orthopedics, China-Japan Friendship Hospital, Beijing, China.
Li X	Shanghai Key Laboratory of New Drug Design, School of Pharmacy, East China University of Science and Technology, 130 Meilong Road, Shanghai 200237, China; Shanghai Institute of Materia Medica, Chinese Academy of Sciences, 555 Zuchongzhi Road, Shanghai 201203, China.; Shanghai Key Laboratory of New Drug Design, School of Pharmacy, East China University of Science and Technology, 130 Meilong Road, Shanghai 200237, China. Electronic address: ytang234@ecust.edu.cn.

Name of Author	Institutional Affiliation
Ouyang L	Sichuan Academy of Medical Science & Sichuan Provincial People's Hospital, School of Medicine of University of Electronic Science and Technology of China, Chinese Academy of Sciences Sichuan Translational Medicine Research Hospital, Chengdu 610072, China.; Sichuan Academy of Medical Science & Sichuan Provincial People's Hospital, School of Medicine of University of Electronic Science and Technology of China, Chinese Academy of Sciences Sichuan Translational Medicine Research Hospital, Chengdu 610072, China; State Key Laboratory of Biotherapy & Cancer Center, West China Hospital, Sichuan University, and Collaborative Innovation Center of Biotherapy, Chengdu 610041, China. Electronic address: shijianyoude@126.com.; State Key Laboratory of Biotherapy & Cancer Center, West China Hospital, Sichuan University, and Collaborative Innovation Center of Biotherapy, Chengdu 610041, China. Electronic address: ouyangliang@scu.edu.cn.
Shi J	Sichuan Academy of Medical Science & Sichuan Provincial People's Hospital, School of Medicine of University of Electronic Science and Technology of China, Chinese Academy of Sciences Sichuan Translational Medicine Research Hospital, Chengdu 610072, China. Electronic address: shijianyoude@126.com.; State Key Laboratory of Biotherapy & Cancer Center, West China Hospital, Sichuan University, Collaborative Innovation Center of Biotherapy, Chengdu 610041, China. Electronic address: yiwenzhang@scu.edu.cn.
Sun B	Department of Functional Neurosurgery, Ruijin Hospital, Shanghai Jiao Tong University School of Medicine, Shanghai, China.

Name of Author	Institutional Affiliation
Tan L	Department of Neurology, Qingdao Municipal Hospital, Nanjing Medical University, Nanjing, China.; Department of Neurology, Qingdao Municipal Hospital, Nanjing Medical University, Nanjing, China Department of Neurology, Qingdao Municipal Hospital, School of Medicine, Qingdao University, Qingdao, China Department of Neurology, Qingdao Municipal Hospital, College of Medicine and Pharmaceutics, Ocean University of China, Qingdao, China.; Department of Epidemiology and Biostatistics, School of Public Health, Nanjing Medical University, Nanjing, China.; Department of Neurology, Qingdao Municipal Hospital, School of Medicine, Qingdao University, Qingdao, China.
Tang Y	Shanghai Key Laboratory of New Drug Design, School of Pharmacy, East China University of Science and Technology, 130 Meilong Road, Shanghai 200237, China; Shanghai Institute of Materia Medica, Chinese Academy of Sciences, 555 Zuchongzhi Road, Shanghai 201203, China.; Shanghai Key Laboratory of New Drug Design, School of Pharmacy, East China University of Science and Technology, 130 Meilong Road, Shanghai 200237, China. Electronic address: ytang234@ecust.edu.cn.
Tao R	aDepartment of Psychological Medicine, Wenzhou Seventh People's Hospital, Wenzhou, Zhejiang bInstitute of Mental Health, Jining Medical University, Jining, Shandong cDepartment of Psychological Medicine, Tianjin Mental Health Center dDepartment of Psychological Medicine, Tianjin Anning Hospital eDepartment of Neurology, Tianjin Medical University General Hospital, Tianjin fDepartment of Psychological Medicine, Chinese PLA (People's Liberation Army) General Hospital gDepartment of Psychological Medicine, General Hospital of Beijing Military Region, Chinese PLA, Beijing, China.

Name of Author	Institutional Affiliation
Wang HF	Department of Neurology, Qingdao Municipal Hospital, Nanjing Medical University, Nanjing, China.; Department of Neurology, Qingdao Municipal Hospital, Nanjing Medical University, Nanjing, China Department of Neurology, Qingdao Municipal Hospital, School of Medicine, Qingdao University, Qingdao, China Department of Neurology, Qingdao Municipal Hospital, College of Medicine and Pharmaceutics, Ocean University of China, Qingdao, China.; Department of Epidemiology and Biostatistics, School of Public Health, Nanjing Medical University, Nanjing, China.; Department of Neurology, Qingdao Municipal Hospital, School of Medicine, Qingdao University, Qingdao, China.
Wei W	College of Integrative Medicine, Fujian University of Traditional Chinese Medicine, Fuzhou, 350122, China. 441000, China. Province, 364000, China. Fuzhou, 350003, China. Medicine, Fuzhou, 350122, China. caij1@163.com.
Xie CL	Department of Neurology, The First Affiliated Hospital of Wenzhou Medical University, Wenzhou, 325000, China. University, Wenzhou, 35000, China. University, Wenzhou, 325000, China. Yuying Children's Hospital of Wenzhou Medical University, Wenzhou, 325027, China. Children's Hospital of Wenzhou Medical University, Wenzhou, 325027, China. 69365560@qq.com. University, Wenzhou, 325000, China. xiechenglong1987@sina.com.
Yu Z	aDepartment of Acupuncture, China-Japan Friendship Hospital, Beijing bDepartment of Neurology, The Affiliated Hospital of Yangzhou University, Yangzhou University, Yangzhou, Jiangsu Province cDepartment of Orthopedics, Tumd Right Banner Hospital, Baotou City dDepartment of Orthopedics, China-Japan Friendship Hospital, Beijing, China.

Name of Author	Institutional Affiliation
Zhang H	Sichuan Academy of Medical Science & Sichuan Provincial People's Hospital, School of Medicine of University of Electronic Science and Technology of China, Chinese Academy of Sciences Sichuan Translational Medicine Research Hospital, Chengdu 610072, China.; Sichuan Academy of Medical Science & Sichuan Provincial People's Hospital, School of Medicine of University of Electronic Science and Technology of China, Chinese Academy of Sciences Sichuan Translational Medicine Research Hospital, Chengdu 610072, China; State Key Laboratory of Biotherapy & Cancer Center, West China Hospital, Sichuan University, and Collaborative Innovation Center of Biotherapy, Chengdu 610041, China. Electronic address: shijianyoude@126.com.; State Key Laboratory of Biotherapy & Cancer Center, West China Hospital, Sichuan University, and Collaborative Innovation Center of Biotherapy, Chengdu 610041, China. Electronic address: ouyangliang@scu.edu.cn.
Zhang TY	From the Departments of Neurology (T-YZ, YH, Z-YN, FC, QG, LZ, L-JJ) and Spine Surgery (R-XJ, BH, C-YG), Shanghai Tongji Hospital, Tongji University School of Medicine, Shanghai, China.
Zhu ZG	Department of Neurology, The First Affiliated Hospital of Wenzhou Medical University, Wenzhou, 325000, China. University, Wenzhou, 35000, China. University, Wenzhou, 325000, China. Yuying Children's Hospital of Wenzhou Medical University, Wenzhou, 325027, China. Children's Hospital of Wenzhou Medical University, Wenzhou, 325027, China. 69365560@qq.com. University, Wenzhou, 325000, China. xiechenglong1987@sina.com.

Name of Author	Institutional Affiliation
Zhuo C	aDepartment of Psychological Medicine, Wenzhou Seventh People's Hospital, Wenzhou, Zhejiang bInstitute of Mental Health, Jining Medical University, Jining, Shandong cDepartment of Psychological Medicine, Tianjin Mental Health Center dDepartment of Psychological Medicine, Tianjin Anning Hospital eDepartment of Neurology, Tianjin Medical University General Hospital, Tianjin fDepartment of Psychological Medicine, Chinese PLA (People's Liberation Army) General Hospital gDepartment of Psychological Medicine, General Hospital of Beijing Military Region, Chinese PLA, Beijing, China.

Croatia

Name of Author	Institutional Affiliation
Bago Rozankovic P	Department of Neurology, University Hospital Dubrava, Avenija Gojka Suska 6, 10000 Zagreb, Croatia. Electronic address: petrabago@yahoo.com. 10000 Zagreb, Croatia. 10000 Zagreb, Croatia. 10000 Zagreb, Croatia.
Stojic M	Department of Neurology, University Hospital Dubrava, Avenija Gojka Suska 6, 10000 Zagreb, Croatia. Electronic address: petrabago@yahoo.com. 10000 Zagreb, Croatia. 10000 Zagreb, Croatia. 10000 Zagreb, Croatia.

Czech Republic

Name of Author	Institutional Affiliation
Kanovsky P	Department of Neurology. Dentistry, Palacky University Olomouc, Czech Republic. in Bratislava and University Hospital in Martin, Slovak Republic. in Bratislava and University Hospital in Martin, Slovak Republic. University Olomouc, Czech Republic.

Name of Author	Institutional Affiliation
Kurcova S	Department of Neurology. Dentistry, Palacky University Olomouc, Czech Republic. in Bratislava and University Hospital in Martin, Slovak Republic. in Bratislava and University Hospital in Martin, Slovak Republic. University Olomouc, Czech Republic.

Finland

Name of Author	Institutional Affiliation
Mertsalmi TH	Department of Neurology, Helsinki University Hospital, Helsinki, Finland. Helsinki, Finland. Helsinki, Helsinki, Finland. Helsinki, Helsinki, Finland. Helsinki, Helsinki, Finland. Helsinki, Finland. Helsinki, Helsinki, Finland.
Scheperjans F	Department of Neurology, Helsinki University Hospital, Helsinki, Finland. Helsinki, Finland. Helsinki, Helsinki, Finland. Helsinki, Helsinki, Finland. Helsinki, Helsinki, Finland. Helsinki, Finland. Helsinki, Helsinki, Finland.
Sihvonen AJ	Faculty of Medicine, University of Turku, Turku, Finland; Cognitive Brain Research Unit, Department of Psychology and Logopedics, Faculty of Medicine, University of Helsinki, Finland. Electronic address: ajsihv@utu.fi. of Medicine, University of Helsinki, Finland. of Medicine, University of Helsinki, Finland. of Medicine, University of Helsinki, Finland; CICERO Learning, University of Helsinki, Finland. Drama Hannover, Hanover, Germany. Clinical Neurosciences, Turku University Hospital, Turku, Finland.
Soinila S	Faculty of Medicine, University of Turku, Turku, Finland; Cognitive Brain Research Unit, Department of Psychology and Logopedics, Faculty of Medicine, University of Helsinki, Finland. Electronic address: ajsihv@utu.fi. of Medicine, University of Helsinki, Finland. of Medicine, University of Helsinki, Finland. of Medicine, University of Helsinki, Finland; CICERO Learning, University of Helsinki, Finland. Drama Hannover, Hanover, Germany. Clinical Neurosciences, Turku University Hospital, Turku, Finland.

France

Name of Author	Institutional Affiliation
Baille G	Department of Neurology and Movement Disorders, Lille University Medical Center, Lille, France. Lille, France. France. Lille, France.
Cury RG	From the Service de Neurologie (R.G.C., V.F., A.C., M.A.P.F., E.M.), Service de Neurochirurgie (M.A.P.F., E.S.), Centre Hospitalier Universitaire de Grenoble, Universite Grenoble Alpes, INSERM U1216, Grenoble, France; Department of Neurology (R.G.C., M.A.P.F., E.J.L.A.), School of Medicine, University of Sao Paulo, Sao Paulo, Brazil; Hospital Dr. Dario Contreras (M.A.P.F.), Santo Domingo, Republica Dominicana; Service de Neurologie (P.K., S.C.), CHU de Geneve, Switzerland; and Clinatec (A.-L.B.), Centre Hospitalier Universitaire de Grenoble, France. elenamfmoro@gmail.com.
Hauser RA	Parkinson's Disease and Movement Disorders Center, University of South Florida, National Parkinson Foundation Center of Excellence, Tampa. Raffaele, Rome, Italy. Medicale, Toulouse University, Toulouse, France.
Hewitt D	Parkinson's Disease and Movement Disorders Center, University of South Florida, National Parkinson Foundation Center of Excellence, Tampa. Raffaele, Rome, Italy. Medicale, Toulouse University, Toulouse, France.
Moreau C	Department of Neurology and Movement Disorders, Lille University Medical Center, Lille, France. Lille, France. France. Lille, France.

Name of Author	Institutional Affiliation
Moro E	From the Service de Neurologie (R.G.C., V.F., A.C., M.A.P.F., E.M.), Service de Neurochirurgie (M.A.P.F., E.S.), Centre Hospitalier Universitaire de Grenoble, Universite Grenoble Alpes, INSERM U1216, Grenoble, France; Department of Neurology (R.G.C., M.A.P.F., E.J.L.A.), School of Medicine, University of Sao Paulo, Sao Paulo, Brazil; Hospital Dr. Dario Contreras (M.A.P.F.), Santo Domingo, Republica Dominicana; Service de Neurologie (P.K., S.C.), CHU de Geneve, Switzerland; and Clinatec (A.-L.B.), Centre Hospitalier Universitaire de Grenoble, France. elenamfmoro@gmail.com.

Germany

Name of Author	Institutional Affiliation
Bussing A	Quality of Life, Spirituality and Coping, Institute of Integrative Medicine, Faculty of Health, University Witten/Herdecke, Herdecke, Germany. desiree.loetzke@uni-wh.de. Herdecke, Germany. desiree.loetzke@uni-wh.de. Herdecke, Germany. thomas.ostermann@uni-wh.de. Witten/Herdecke, Herdecke, Germany. thomas.ostermann@uni-wh.de. Faculty of Health, University Witten/Herdecke, Herdecke, Germany. arndt.buessing@uni-wh.de. Herdecke, Germany. arndt.buessing@uni-wh.de.
Hopp M	Paracelsus-Elena Hospital, Kassel, Germany; Department of Neurosurgery, University Medical Centre, Goettingen, Germany. Electronic address: ctrenkwalder@gmx.de. Hospital, London, UK; Biomedical Research Unit for Dementia, King's College, London, UK. Hospital, Toulouse, France. Faculty of Medicine in Hradec Kralove and University Hospital Hradec Kralove, Hradec Kralove, Czech Republic. Hospital Clinic, CIBERNED, Barcelona, Spain. Witten/Herdecke, Faculty of Health, Witten, Germany. Pharmacology, Justus-Liebig-Universitat Giessen, Germany.

Name of Author	Institutional Affiliation
Kalenscher T	Comparative Psychology, Institute of Experimental Psychology, Heinrich-Heine University Dusseldorf , 40225 Dusseldorf, Germany.; Institute of Clinical Neuroscience and Medical Psychology, Medical Faculty, Heinrich-Heine University Dusseldorf , 40225 Dusseldorf, Germany.
Klingelhoefer L	Department of Neurology, Technical University Dresden, Dresden, Germany.
Li K	a 1 Center of Clinical Neuroscience, Technical University Dresden, Dresden, Germany.
Lotzke D	Quality of Life, Spirituality and Coping, Institute of Integrative Medicine, Faculty of Health, University Witten/Herdecke, Herdecke, Germany. desiree.loetzke@uni-wh.de. Herdecke, Germany. desiree.loetzke@uni-wh.de. Herdecke, Germany. thomas.ostermann@uni-wh.de. Witten/Herdecke, Herdecke, Germany. thomas.ostermann@uni-wh.de. Faculty of Health, University Witten/Herdecke, Herdecke, Germany. arndt.buessing@uni-wh.de. Herdecke, Germany. arndt.buessing@uni-wh.de.
Muller T	Department of Neurology, St. Joseph Hospital Berlin-Weissensee, Berlin, Germany. thomas.mueller@ruhr-uni-bochum.de.
Odin P	aDepartment of Clinical Sciences Lund, Faculty of Medicine, Lund University bDepartment of Neurology, Skane University Hospital, Lund, Sweden cDepartment of Neurology, Central Hospital, Bremerhaven, Germany.
Reichmann H	Department of Neurology, Technical University Dresden, Dresden, Germany.
Seinstra M	Comparative Psychology, Institute of Experimental Psychology, Heinrich-Heine University Dusseldorf , 40225 Dusseldorf, Germany.; Institute of Clinical Neuroscience and Medical Psychology, Medical Faculty, Heinrich-Heine University Dusseldorf , 40225 Dusseldorf, Germany.

Name of Author	Institutional Affiliation
Timpka J	aDepartment of Clinical Sciences Lund, Faculty of Medicine, Lund University bDepartment of Neurology, Skane University Hospital, Lund, Sweden cDepartment of Neurology, Central Hospital, Bremerhaven, Germany.
Trenkwalder C	Paracelsus-Elena Hospital, Kassel, Germany; Department of Neurosurgery, University Medical Centre, Goettingen, Germany. Electronic address: ctrenkwalder@gmx.de. Hospital, London, UK; Biomedical Research Unit for Dementia, King's College, London, UK. Hospital, Toulouse, France. Faculty of Medicine in Hradec Kralove and University Hospital Hradec Kralove, Hradec Kralove, Czech Republic. Hospital Clinic, CIBERNED, Barcelona, Spain. Witten/Herdecke, Faculty of Health, Witten, Germany. Pharmacology, Justus-Liebig-Universitat Giessen, Germany.
Ziemssen T	a 1 Center of Clinical Neuroscience, Technical University Dresden, Dresden, Germany.

Hungary

Name of Author	Institutional Affiliation
Annus A	Department of Neurology, Faculty of Medicine, Albert Szent-Gyorgyi Clinical Center, University of Szeged. Center, University of Szeged; MTA-SZTE Neuroscience Research Group, Szeged, Hungary.
Vecsei L	Department of Neurology, Faculty of Medicine, Albert Szent-Gyorgyi Clinical Center, University of Szeged. Center, University of Szeged; MTA-SZTE Neuroscience Research Group, Szeged, Hungary.

India

Name of Author	Institutional Affiliation
Pathak-Gandhi N	Medical Research Centre - Kasturba Health Society, 17 K Desai Road, Mumbai, India. Electronic address: namyata@gmail.com. India. Electronic address: ashokdbv@gmail.com.
Vaidya AD	Medical Research Centre - Kasturba Health Society, 17 K Desai Road, Mumbai, India. Electronic address: namyata@gmail.com. India. Electronic address: ashokdbv@gmail.com.

Ireland

Name of Author	Institutional Affiliation
Clifford AM	Faculty of Education and Health Sciences, Department of Clinical Therapies, University of Limerick, Limerick, Ireland. Electronic address: joanne.s@outlook.com. Bundoora, Victoria, Australia. and Dance, University of Limerick, Limerick, Ireland. Limerick, Limerick, Ireland. University of Limerick, Limerick, Ireland.
Shanahan J	Faculty of Education and Health Sciences, Department of Clinical Therapies, University of Limerick, Limerick, Ireland. Electronic address: joanne.s@outlook.com. Bundoora, Victoria, Australia. and Dance, University of Limerick, Limerick, Ireland. Limerick, Limerick, Ireland. University of Limerick, Limerick, Ireland.

Israel

Name of Author	Institutional Affiliation
Balash Y	*Movement Disorders Unit, Neurological Institute, Tel Aviv Sourasky Medical Center, Tel Aviv; daggerSackler School of Medicine, Tel Aviv University, Tel Aviv; double daggerTikun Olam, Research Department, Tel Aviv; section signSchool of Public Health, Epidemiology, Sackler School of Medicine, Tel-Aviv University, Tel-Aviv; parallelOneWorld Cannabis Ltd, Petah-Tikva; paragraph signMovement Disorders Center, Rabin Medical Center, Petah-Tikva; and #Sagol School of Neuroscience, Tel Aviv University, Tel Aviv, Israel.
Bergman J	*Mental Health Center, Ma'ale Carmel, The Ruth and Bruce Rappaport Faculty of Medicine, Technion, Haifa; daggerGeha Mental Health Center, Petakh Tikva; double daggerIsrael Defense Force, Tel Aviv; and section signBe'er-Sheva Mental Health Center, Faculty of Health Sciences, Ben-Gurion University of the Negev, Be'er-Sheva, Israel.
Gurevich T	*Movement Disorders Unit, Neurological Institute, Tel Aviv Sourasky Medical Center, Tel Aviv; daggerSackler School of Medicine, Tel Aviv University, Tel Aviv; double daggerTikun Olam, Research Department, Tel Aviv; section signSchool of Public Health, Epidemiology, Sackler School of Medicine, Tel-Aviv University, Tel-Aviv; parallelOneWorld Cannabis Ltd, Petah-Tikva; paragraph signMovement Disorders Center, Rabin Medical Center, Petah-Tikva; and #Sagol School of Neuroscience, Tel Aviv University, Tel Aviv, Israel.
Miodownik C	*Mental Health Center, Ma'ale Carmel, The Ruth and Bruce Rappaport Faculty of Medicine, Technion, Haifa; daggerGeha Mental Health Center, Petakh Tikva; double daggerIsrael Defense Force, Tel Aviv; and section signBe'er-Sheva Mental Health Center, Faculty of Health Sciences, Ben-Gurion University of the Negev, Be'er-Sheva, Israel.

Italy

Name of Author	Institutional Affiliation
Allone C	Department of Clinical Neurosciences and Neurobioimaging. Istituto di Ricovero e Cura a Carattere Scientifico, Centro Neurolesi 'Bonino-Pulejo' Messina, Messina, Italy.; Department of Biomedical and Dental Sciences and Morphological and Functional Imaging, University of Messina, Messina, Italy.
Antonini A	Department of Neurology, Azienda Ospedaliera Universitaria Arcispedale S.Anna, Ferrara, Italy. giovannicossu@aob.it. Arcugnano, Vicenza, Italy. Turin, Italy.
Biundo R	Parkinson's Disease and Movement Disorders Unit, San Camillo Hospital IRCCS, Venice, Italy. Venice, Italy. Venice, Italy. Venice, Italy.
De Virgilio A	Department Organs of Sense, ENT Section, 'Sapienza' University of Rome, Viale del Policlinico 155, 00100, Rome, Italy; Department of Surgical Science, 'Sapienza' University of Rome, Viale del Policlinico 155, 00100, Rome, Italy. Electronic address: mariaidarizzo@gmail.com.; Department Organs of Sense, ENT Section, 'Sapienza' University of Rome, Viale del Policlinico 155, 00100, Rome, Italy.; Department of Neurology and Psychiatry, 'Sapienza' University of Rome, Viale del Policlinico 155, 00100, Rome, Italy.; Department of Medico-Surgical Sciences and Biotechnologies, Otorhinolaryngology Section, 'Sapienza' University of Rome, Corso della Repubblica, 79, 04100 Latina, Italy.
Deriu F	Department of Biomedical Sciences, University of Sassari, Sassari, Italy. Italy. Sassari, Italy. Sassari, Italy. Sassari, Italy.

Name of Author	Institutional Affiliation
Frazzitta G	Department of Parkinson Disease and Brain Injury Rehabilitation, 'Moriggia-Pelascini' Hospital, Gravedona ed Uniti, Italy. Electronic address: grazia.palamara@gmail.com.; Department of Biomedical Engineering, Scientific Institute of Montescano, S. Maugeri Foundation IRCCS, Montescano, Italy.; Department of Physical Medicine and Rehabilitation, S. Raffaele Arcangelo Fatebenefratelli Hospital, Venice, Italy.
Geroin C	Neuromotor and Cognitive Rehabilitation Research Center (CRRNC), Department of Neurological, Biomedical and Movement Sciences, University of Verona, P.le L.A. Scuro 10, 37134, Verona, Italy. christian.geroin@univr.it. Neurological, Biomedical and Movement Sciences, University of Verona, P.le L.A. Scuro 10, 37134, Verona, Italy. marialuisa.gandolfi@univr.it. 10, 37134, Verona, Italy. marialuisa.gandolfi@univr.it. Program in Parkinson's Disease, Toronto Western Hospital, University Health Network, Toronto, ON, Canada. veubru@gmail.com. Neurological, Biomedical and Movement Sciences, University of Verona, P.le L.A. Scuro 10, 37134, Verona, Italy. nicola.smania@univr.it. 10, 37134, Verona, Italy. nicola.smania@univr.it. Biomedical and Movement Sciences, University of Verona, P.le Scuro 10, 37134, Verona, Italy. michele.tinazzi@univr.it.
Lavano A	Department of Neurosurgery, "Magna Graecia" University, Catanzaro, Italy - lavano@unicz.it.
Lopiano L	Department of Neurology, Gardner Family Center for Parkinson's Disease and Movement Disorders, University of Cincinnati (UC), 260 Stetson Street, Suite 4244, Cincinnati, OH, 45219, USA. merolaae@ucmail.uc.edu.; Department of Neuroscience 'Rita Levi Montalcini', University of Turin, via Cherasco 15, 10124, Turin, Italy.; Department of Neurosurgery, Neuroscience Institute and UC College of Medicine, University of Cincinnati (UC), Cincinnati, OH, USA.

Name of Author	Institutional Affiliation
Marino S	Department of Clinical Neurosciences and Neurobioimaging. Istituto di Ricovero e Cura a Carattere Scientifico, Centro Neurolesi 'Bonino-Pulejo' Messina, Messina, Italy.; Department of Biomedical and Dental Sciences and Morphological and Functional Imaging, University of Messina, Messina, Italy.
Merola A	Department of Neurology, Gardner Family Center for Parkinson's Disease and Movement Disorders, University of Cincinnati (UC), 260 Stetson Street, Suite 4244, Cincinnati, OH, 45219, USA. merolaae@ucmail.uc.edu.; Department of Neuroscience 'Rita Levi Montalcini', University of Turin, via Cherasco 15, 10124, Turin, Italy.; Department of Neurosurgery, Neuroscience Institute and UC College of Medicine, University of Cincinnati (UC), Cincinnati, OH, USA.
Mostile G	Dipartimento "G.F. Ingrassia", Sezione di Neuroscienze, Universita Degli Studi di Catania, Catania, Italy.
Nicoletti A	Department "G.F. Ingrassia", Section of Neurosciences, University of Catania, Catania, Italy. Catania, Italy. Genoa, Genoa, Italy. Italy. Palermo, Palermo, Italy. Institute, Cassino (FR), Italy. University of Rome, Rome, Italy. Institute C. Mondino, Pavia, Italy. Second University of Naples, Naples, Italy.
Palamara G	Department of Parkinson Disease and Brain Injury Rehabilitation, 'Moriggia-Pelascini' Hospital, Gravedona ed Uniti, Italy. Electronic address: grazia.palamara@gmail.com.; Department of Biomedical Engineering, Scientific Institute of Montescano, S. Maugeri Foundation IRCCS, Montescano, Italy.; Department of Physical Medicine and Rehabilitation, S. Raffaele Arcangelo Fatebenefratelli Hospital, Venice, Italy.
Sensi M	Department of Neurology, Azienda Ospedaliera Universitaria Arcispedale S.Anna, Ferrara, Italy. giovannicossu@aob.it. Arcugnano, Vicenza, Italy. Turin, Italy.

Name of Author	Institutional Affiliation
Tinazzi M	Neuromotor and Cognitive Rehabilitation Research Center (CRRNC), Department of Neurological, Biomedical and Movement Sciences, University of Verona, P.le L.A. Scuro 10, 37134, Verona, Italy. christian.geroin@univr.it. Neurological, Biomedical and Movement Sciences, University of Verona, P.le L.A. Scuro 10, 37134, Verona, Italy. marialuisa.gandolfi@univr.it. 10, 37134, Verona, Italy. marialuisa.gandolfi@univr.it. Program in Parkinson's Disease, Toronto Western Hospital, University Health Network, Toronto, ON, Canada. veubru@gmail.com. Neurological, Biomedical and Movement Sciences, University of Verona, P.le L.A. Scuro 10, 37134, Verona, Italy. nicola.smania@univr.it. 10, 37134, Verona, Italy. nicola.smania@univr.it. Biomedical and Movement Sciences, University of Verona, P.le Scuro 10, 37134, Verona, Italy. michele.tinazzi@univr.it.
Volpentesta G	Department of Neurosurgery, "Magna Graecia" University, Catanzaro, Italy - lavano@unicz.it.
Zappia M	Department "G.F. Ingrassia", Section of Neurosciences, University of Catania, Catania, Italy. Catania, Italy. Genoa, Genoa, Italy. Italy. Palermo, Palermo, Italy. Institute, Cassino (FR), Italy. University of Rome, Rome, Italy. Institute C. Mondino, Pavia, Italy. Second University of Naples, Naples, Italy.
de Natale ER	Department of Biomedical Sciences, University of Sassari, Sassari, Italy. Italy. Sassari, Italy. Sassari, Italy. Sassari, Italy.

Name of Author	Institutional Affiliation
de Vincentiis M	Department Organs of Sense, ENT Section, 'Sapienza' University of Rome, Viale del Policlinico 155, 00100, Rome, Italy; Department of Surgical Science, 'Sapienza' University of Rome, Viale del Policlinico 155, 00100, Rome, Italy. Electronic address: mariaidarizzo@gmail.com.; Department Organs of Sense, ENT Section, 'Sapienza' University of Rome, Viale del Policlinico 155, 00100, Rome, Italy.; Department of Neurology and Psychiatry, 'Sapienza' University of Rome, Viale del Policlinico 155, 00100, Rome, Italy.; Department of Medico-Surgical Sciences and Biotechnologies, Otorhinolaryngology Section, 'Sapienza' University of Rome, Corso della Repubblica, 79, 04100 Latina, Italy.

Japan

Name of Author	Institutional Affiliation
Barker RA	Department of Clinical Neuroscience and Cambridge Stem Cell Institute, Forvie Site, Cambridge CB2 0PY, UK. Lund Stem Cell Centre, Department of Experimental Medical Science, Lund University, 22184, Lund, Sweden. Electronic address: malin.parmar@med.lu.se. Cancer Center, New York, NY 10022, USA. Kyoto University, 606-8507, Kyoto, Japan.
Bhidayasiri R	Chulalongkorn Center of Excellence for Parkinson Disease & Related Disorders, Department of Medicine, Faculty of Medicine, Chulalongkorn University, King Chulalongkorn Memorial Hospital, Thai Red Cross Society, Bangkok, 10330, Thailand.; Chulalongkorn Center of Excellence for Parkinson Disease & Related Disorders, Department of Medicine, Faculty of Medicine, Chulalongkorn University, King Chulalongkorn Memorial Hospital, Thai Red Cross Society, Bangkok, 10330, Thailand; Department of Rehabilitation Medicine, Juntendo University, Tokyo, Japan. Electronic address: rbh@chulapd.org.

Name of Author	Institutional Affiliation
Foongsathaporn C	Chulalongkorn Center of Excellence for Parkinson Disease & Related Disorders, Department of Medicine, Faculty of Medicine, Chulalongkorn University, King Chulalongkorn Memorial Hospital, Thai Red Cross Society, Bangkok, 10330, Thailand.; Chulalongkorn Center of Excellence for Parkinson Disease & Related Disorders, Department of Medicine, Faculty of Medicine, Chulalongkorn University, King Chulalongkorn Memorial Hospital, Thai Red Cross Society, Bangkok, 10330, Thailand; Department of Rehabilitation Medicine, Juntendo University, Tokyo, Japan. Electronic address: rbh@chulapd.org.
Hirato M	Department of Neurosurgery, Gunma University Graduate School of Medicine, Maebashi, Gunma, Japan. Electronic address: mfhirato@gunma-u.ac.jp. Maebashi, Gunma, Japan. Maebashi, Gunma, Japan.
Maeda T	Division of Neurology and Gerontology, Department of Internal Medicine, School of Medicine, Iwate Medical University, 19-1 Uchimaru, Morioka, Iwate 020-8505, Japan; Department of Neurology and Movement Disorder Research, Research Institute for Brain and Blood Vessels-Akita, 6-10 Senshukubotamachi, Akita 010-0874, Japan. Electronic address: maeda@iwate-med.ac.jp.; Department of Neurology, Juntendo University School of Medicine 3-1-3 Hongo, Bunkyo-ku, Tokyo 113-8431, Japan. Electronic address: yshimo@juntendo.ac.jp.; Division of Biostatistics, Tohoku University Graduate School of Medicine, 2-1 Seiryo-machi, Aoba-ku, Sendai, Miyagi, 980-8575, Japan. Electronic address: chiu@med.tohoku.ac.jp.; Division of Biostatistics, Tohoku University Graduate School of Medicine, 2-1 Seiryo-machi, Aoba-ku, Sendai, Miyagi, 980-8575, Japan. Electronic address: yamaguchi@med.tohoku.ac.jp.; Department of Neurology, Okayama Kyokuto Hospital, 567-1 Kurata, Okayama, 703-8265, Japan. Electronic address: kkashi@kyokuto.or.jp.

Name of Author	Institutional Affiliation
Saiki H	Division of Neurology and Gerontology, Department of Internal Medicine, School of Medicine, Iwate Medical University, 19-1 Uchimaru, Morioka, Iwate 020-8505, Japan; Department of Neurology and Movement Disorder Research, Research Institute for Brain and Blood Vessels-Akita, 6-10 Senshukubotamachi, Akita 010-0874, Japan. Electronic address: maeda@iwate-med.ac.jp.; Department of Neurology, Juntendo University School of Medicine 3-1-3 Hongo, Bunkyo-ku, Tokyo 113-8431, Japan. Electronic address: yshimo@juntendo.ac.jp.; Division of Biostatistics, Tohoku University Graduate School of Medicine, 2-1 Seiryo-machi, Aoba-ku, Sendai, Miyagi, 980-8575, Japan. Electronic address: chiu@med.tohoku.ac.jp.; Division of Biostatistics, Tohoku University Graduate School of Medicine, 2-1 Seiryo-machi, Aoba-ku, Sendai, Miyagi, 980-8575, Japan. Electronic address: yamaguchi@med.tohoku.ac.jp.; Department of Neurology, Okayama Kyokuto Hospital, 567-1 Kurata, Okayama, 703-8265, Japan. Electronic address: kkashi@kyokuto.or.jp.
Sasaki H	*Department of Neurology, Faculty of Medicine and Graduate School of Medicine, Hokkaido University; and daggerDepartment of Neurology, Sapporo Teishinkai Hospital, Sapporo, Japan.
Takahashi J	Department of Clinical Neuroscience and Cambridge Stem Cell Institute, Forvie Site, Cambridge CB2 0PY, UK. Lund Stem Cell Centre, Department of Experimental Medical Science, Lund University, 22184, Lund, Sweden. Electronic address: malin.parmar@med.lu.se. Cancer Center, New York, NY 10022, USA. Kyoto University, 606-8507, Kyoto, Japan.
Yabe I	*Department of Neurology, Faculty of Medicine and Graduate School of Medicine, Hokkaido University; and daggerDepartment of Neurology, Sapporo Teishinkai Hospital, Sapporo, Japan.

Name of Author	Institutional Affiliation
Yoshimoto Y	Department of Neurosurgery, Gunma University Graduate School of Medicine, Maebashi, Gunma, Japan. Electronic address: mfhirato@gunma-u.ac.jp. Maebashi, Gunma, Japan. Maebashi, Gunma, Japan.

Korea

Name of Author	Institutional Affiliation
Cho SY	1 Department of Cardiology and Neurology, College of Korean Medicine, Kyung Hee University , Seoul, Republic of Korea.; 2 Stroke and Neurological Disorders Center, Kyung Hee University Hospital at Gangdong , Seoul, Republic of Korea.; 3 Department of Epidemiology and Biostatistics, Graduate School of Public Health and Institute of Health and Environment, Seoul University , Seoul, Republic of Korea.; 4 Department of Neurology, Kyung Hee University Hospital at Gangdong, College of Medicine, Kyung Hee University , Seoul, Republic of Korea.; 5 Integrative Parkinson's Disease Research Group, Acupuncture and Meridian Science Research Center, Kyung Hee University , Seoul, Republic of Korea.
Lee J	1 Yonsei University, Seodaemun-gu, Seoul, Korea.
Lee SH	aDepartment of Applied Korean Medicine, College of Korean Medicine, Graduate School, Kyung Hee University bResearch Group of Pain and Neuroscience, WHO Collaborating Center for Traditional Medicine, East-West Medical Research Institute cDepartment of Meridian and Acupoint, College of Korean Medicine, Kyung Hee University, Seoul, Republic of Korea.
Lim S	aDepartment of Applied Korean Medicine, College of Korean Medicine, Graduate School, Kyung Hee University bResearch Group of Pain and Neuroscience, WHO Collaborating Center for Traditional Medicine, East-West Medical Research Institute cDepartment of Meridian and Acupoint, College of Korean Medicine, Kyung Hee University, Seoul, Republic of Korea.

Name of Author	Institutional Affiliation
Park SU	1 Department of Cardiology and Neurology, College of Korean Medicine, Kyung Hee University , Seoul, Republic of Korea.; 2 Stroke and Neurological Disorders Center, Kyung Hee University Hospital at Gangdong , Seoul, Republic of Korea.; 3 Department of Epidemiology and Biostatistics, Graduate School of Public Health and Institute of Health and Environment, Seoul University , Seoul, Republic of Korea.; 4 Department of Neurology, Kyung Hee University Hospital at Gangdong, College of Medicine, Kyung Hee University , Seoul, Republic of Korea.; 5 Integrative Parkinson's Disease Research Group, Acupuncture and Meridian Science Research Center, Kyung Hee University , Seoul, Republic of Korea.
Yoo Y	1 Yonsei University, Seodaemun-gu, Seoul, Korea.

Malaysia

Name of Author	Institutional Affiliation
Amro MS	Department of Anatomy, Universiti Kebangsaan Malaysia Medical Centre, 56000 Kuala Lumpur, Malaysia. Lumpur, Malaysia. Lumpur, Malaysia. Lumpur, Malaysia.
Srijit D	Department of Anatomy, Universiti Kebangsaan Malaysia Medical Centre, 56000 Kuala Lumpur, Malaysia. Lumpur, Malaysia. Lumpur, Malaysia. Lumpur, Malaysia.

Mexico

Name of Author	Institutional Affiliation
Corona T	Unidad de Investigacion de Enfermedades Neurodegenerativas Clinicas, Instituto Nacional de Neurologia y Neurocirugia, Ciudad de Mexico, Mexico; Clinica de Trastornos del Movimiento, Instituto Nacional de Neurologia y Neurocirugia, Ciudad de Mexico, Mexico.; Unidad de Investigacion de Enfermedades Neurodegenerativas Clinicas, Instituto Nacional de Neurologia y Neurocirugia, Ciudad de Mexico, Mexico. Electronic address: coronav@unam.mx.
Rodriguez-Violante M	Unidad de Investigacion de Enfermedades Neurodegenerativas Clinicas, Instituto Nacional de Neurologia y Neurocirugia, Ciudad de Mexico, Mexico; Clinica de Trastornos del Movimiento, Instituto Nacional de Neurologia y Neurocirugia, Ciudad de Mexico, Mexico.; Unidad de Investigacion de Enfermedades Neurodegenerativas Clinicas, Instituto Nacional de Neurologia y Neurocirugia, Ciudad de Mexico, Mexico. Electronic address: coronav@unam.mx.

Netherlands

Name of Author	Institutional Affiliation
Elbers RG	Department of Physiotherapy, University of Applied Sciences, Leiden, the Netherlands2Department of Rehabilitation Medicine, VU University Medical Center, Amsterdam, the Netherlands. Netherlands. the Netherlands.
Kwakkel G	Department of Physiotherapy, University of Applied Sciences, Leiden, the Netherlands2Department of Rehabilitation Medicine, VU University Medical Center, Amsterdam, the Netherlands. Netherlands. the Netherlands.

Norway

Name of Author	Institutional Affiliation
Alves G	From the Norwegian Centre for Movement Disorders (K.F.P., G.A.); Department of Neurology (K.F.P., G.A.) and Memory Clinic (K.F.P., G.A.), Stavanger University Hospital; Network for Medical Sciences (J.P.L.), University of Stavanger; and Department of Neurology (O.-B.T.), Haukeland University Hospital, Bergen, Norway. pekf@sus.no.
Brakedal B	Department of Neurology, Haukeland University Hospital, Bergen, Norway.
Larsen JP	The Norwegian Centre for Movement Disorders, Stavanger University Hospital, Stavanger, Norway. Stavanger, Norway. Stavanger, Norway. Stavanger, Norway. Stavanger, Norway.
Lilleeng B	The Norwegian Centre for Movement Disorders, Stavanger University Hospital, Stavanger, Norway. Stavanger, Norway. Stavanger, Norway. Stavanger, Norway. Stavanger, Norway.
Pedersen KF	From the Norwegian Centre for Movement Disorders (K.F.P., G.A.); Department of Neurology (K.F.P., G.A.) and Memory Clinic (K.F.P., G.A.), Stavanger University Hospital; Network for Medical Sciences (J.P.L.), University of Stavanger; and Department of Neurology (O.-B.T.), Haukeland University Hospital, Bergen, Norway. pekf@sus.no.
Tzoulis C	Department of Neurology, Haukeland University Hospital, Bergen, Norway.

Pakistan

Name of Author	Institutional Affiliation
Khan MA	Dow Medical College, Dow University of Health Sciences, Karachi, Pakistan.
Tohid H	Dow Medical College, Dow University of Health Sciences, Karachi, Pakistan.

Poland

Name of Author	Institutional Affiliation
Bauer L	Parkinson's Disease and Movement Disorders Center, USF Health - Byrd Institute, National Parkinson Foundation Center of Excellence, Tampa, FL, USA. rhauser@health.usf.edu. Department of Neurology, St Adalbert Hospital, Gdansk, Poland.
Hauser RA	Parkinson's Disease and Movement Disorders Center, USF Health - Byrd Institute, National Parkinson Foundation Center of Excellence, Tampa, FL, USA. rhauser@health.usf.edu. Department of Neurology, St Adalbert Hospital, Gdansk, Poland.

Portugal

Name of Author	Institutional Affiliation
Ferreira JJ	a Laboratory of Clinical Pharmacology and Therapeutics, Faculty of Medicine , University of Lisbon , Lisboa , Portugal. Medicine , University of Lisbon , Lisbon , Portugal. , London , UK. University of Lisbon , Lisboa , Portugal. Medicine , University of Lisbon , Lisbon , Portugal.

Name of Author	Institutional Affiliation
Lees AJ	Reta Lila Weston Institute, University College London, London, England. Recherche Medicale (INSERM) and University Hospital of Toulouse, Toulouse, France4Department of Neurosciences, INSERM and University Hospital of Toulouse, Toulouse, France. Coronado, Portugal. Coronado, Portugal8Department of Pharmacology and Therapeutics, University Porto, Porto, Portugal.
Rodrigues FB	a Laboratory of Clinical Pharmacology and Therapeutics, Faculty of Medicine , University of Lisbon , Lisboa , Portugal. Medicine , University of Lisbon , Lisbon , Portugal. , London , UK. University of Lisbon , Lisboa , Portugal. Medicine , University of Lisbon , Lisbon , Portugal.
Soares-da-Silva P	Reta Lila Weston Institute, University College London, London, England. Recherche Medicale (INSERM) and University Hospital of Toulouse, Toulouse, France4Department of Neurosciences, INSERM and University Hospital of Toulouse, Toulouse, France. Coronado, Portugal. Coronado, Portugal8Department of Pharmacology and Therapeutics, University Porto, Porto, Portugal.

Serbia

Name of Author	Institutional Affiliation
Kostic V	a Clinic of Neurology, Clinical Center of Serbia, Faculty of Medicine , University of Belgrade , Belgrade , Serbia.; b Clinic of Neurology , Clinical Center of Serbia , Belgrade , Serbia.
Svetel M	a Clinic of Neurology, Clinical Center of Serbia, Faculty of Medicine , University of Belgrade , Belgrade , Serbia.; b Clinic of Neurology , Clinical Center of Serbia , Belgrade , Serbia.

Singapore

Name of Author	Institutional Affiliation
Chai CL	Institute of Chemical and Engineering Sciences , A* STAR (Agency of Science, Technology and Research), 8 Biomedical Grove, Neuros #07-01, Singapore 138665, Singapore.
Huleatt PB	Institute of Chemical and Engineering Sciences , A* STAR (Agency of Science, Technology and Research), 8 Biomedical Grove, Neuros #07-01, Singapore 138665, Singapore.
Oosterveld LP	From the Department of Neurology (L.P.O., E.Y.L.N., S.-H.S., K.-Y.T., W.-L.A., E.-K.T., L.C.S.T.), Parkinson's Disease and Movement Disorders Centre, USA National Parkinson Foundation Centre of Excellence, National Neuroscience Institute; and Duke-NUS Graduate Medical School (J.C.A., W.-L.A., E.-K.T., L.C.S.T.), Singapore. louis_tan@nni.com.sg.
Tan LC	From the Department of Neurology (L.P.O., E.Y.L.N., S.-H.S., K.-Y.T., W.-L.A., E.-K.T., L.C.S.T.), Parkinson's Disease and Movement Disorders Centre, USA National Parkinson Foundation Centre of Excellence, National Neuroscience Institute; and Duke-NUS Graduate Medical School (J.C.A., W.-L.A., E.-K.T., L.C.S.T.), Singapore. louis_tan@nni.com.sg.

Spain

Name of Author	Institutional Affiliation
Anand R	Department of Clinical Neurosciences, University College London Institute of Neurology, London, United Kingdom. University of Toronto, Toronto, Ontario, Canada. Universitat Oberta de Catalunya, Barcelona, Spain.
Balestrino R	Department of Neuroscience "Rita Levi Montalcini", University of Turin, Via Cherasco 15, 10124 Torino, Italy. Madrid, Spain. Electronic address: pmartinez@isciii.es.

Name of Author	Institutional Affiliation
Bermudez Torres M	Section of Neurology, Complejo Hospitalario Universitario de Ferrol (CHUF), Hospital A. Marcide, Ferrol, A Coruna, Spain. Electronic address: diegosangar@yahoo.es.; Department of Psychiatry, Complejo Hospitalario Universitario de Ferrol (CHUF), Hospital Naval, Ferrol, A Coruna, Spain.; Department of Family Medicine, Complejo Hospitalario Universitario de Ferrol (CHUF), Ferrol, A Coruna, Spain.
Cacabelos R	EuroEspes Biomedical Research Center, Institute of Medical Science and Genomic Medicine, 15165-Bergondo, Corunna, Spain. rcacabelos@euroespes.com.
Martinez-Martin P	Department of Neuroscience "Rita Levi Montalcini", University of Turin, Via Cherasco 15, 10124 Torino, Italy. Madrid, Spain. Electronic address: pmartinez@isciii.es.
Nunez-Arias D	1 Section of Neurology, Hospital Arquitecto Marcide/Hospital Naval, Complexo Hospitalario Universitario de Ferrol (CHUF), Ferrol, A Coruna, Spain.; 2 Department of Biochemistry and Molecular Biology, Boston University, Boston, MA, USA.; 3 Department of Psychiatry, Hospital Naval, Complexo Hospitalario Universitario de Ferrol (CHUF), Ferrol, A Coruna, Spain.
Santos Garcia D	Section of Neurology, Complejo Hospitalario Universitario de Ferrol (CHUF), Hospital A. Marcide, Ferrol, A Coruna, Spain. Electronic address: diegosangar@yahoo.es.; Department of Psychiatry, Complejo Hospitalario Universitario de Ferrol (CHUF), Hospital Naval, Ferrol, A Coruna, Spain.; Department of Family Medicine, Complejo Hospitalario Universitario de Ferrol (CHUF), Ferrol, A Coruna, Spain.
Santos-Garcia D	1 Section of Neurology, Hospital Arquitecto Marcide/Hospital Naval, Complexo Hospitalario Universitario de Ferrol (CHUF), Ferrol, A Coruna, Spain.; 2 Department of Biochemistry and Molecular Biology, Boston University, Boston, MA, USA.; 3 Department of Psychiatry, Hospital Naval, Complexo Hospitalario Universitario de Ferrol (CHUF), Ferrol, A Coruna, Spain.

Name of Author	Institutional Affiliation
Schapira AH	Department of Clinical Neurosciences, University College London Institute of Neurology, London, United Kingdom. University of Toronto, Toronto, Ontario, Canada. Universitat Oberta de Catalunya, Barcelona, Spain.

Sweden

Name of Author	Institutional Affiliation
Bergquist F	Department of Neurology, Institute of Neuroscience and Physiology at Sahlgrenska Academy, University of Gothenburg, Sahlgrenska University Hospital, 413 45 Goteborg, Sweden. Electronic address: Radu.Constantinescu@vgregion.se.; Department of Neurology, Norra Alvsborgs Lanssjukhus, Sjukhuskansliet, 461 85 Trollhattan, Sweden.; Department of Neuropsychiatry, Minnesmottagningen, Wallinsgatan 6, 431 41 Molndal, Sweden.
Cenci MA	Basal Ganglia Pathophysiology Unit, Department of Experimental Medical Science, Lund University, Lund, Sweden. Electronic address: Veronica.Francardo@med.lu.se. Center: Division of Molecular Therapeutics, New York State Psychiatric Institute, New York 10032, NY, USA. Center: Division of Molecular Therapeutics, New York State Psychiatric Institute, New York 10032, NY, USA. Lund University, Lund, Sweden. Electronic address: Angela.Cenci_Nilsson@med.lu.se.
Constantinescu R	Department of Neurology, Institute of Neuroscience and Physiology at Sahlgrenska Academy, University of Gothenburg, Sahlgrenska University Hospital, 413 45 Goteborg, Sweden. Electronic address: Radu.Constantinescu@vgregion.se.; Department of Neurology, Norra Alvsborgs Lanssjukhus, Sjukhuskansliet, 461 85 Trollhattan, Sweden.; Department of Neuropsychiatry, Minnesmottagningen, Wallinsgatan 6, 431 41 Molndal, Sweden.

Name of Author	Institutional Affiliation
Francardo V	Basal Ganglia Pathophysiology Unit, Department of Experimental Medical Science, Lund University, Lund, Sweden. Electronic address: Veronica.Francardo@med.lu.se. Center: Division of Molecular Therapeutics, New York State Psychiatric Institute, New York 10032, NY, USA. Center: Division of Molecular Therapeutics, New York State Psychiatric Institute, New York 10032, NY, USA. Lund University, Lund, Sweden. Electronic address: Angela.Cenci_Nilsson@med.lu.se.
Hall S	From the Department of Neurology (S.H., Y.S.) and Memory Clinic (O.H.), Skane University Hospital; Department of Clinical Sciences (S.H., Y.S., D.L., O.H.), Lund University; Department of Psychiatry and Neurochemistry (A.O., H.Z.), Institute of Neuroscience and Physiology, the Sahlgrenska Academy at the University of Gothenburg, Gothenburg and Molndal, Sweden; UCL Institute of Neurology (H.Z.), Queen Square, London, UK; and Psychiatry Skane (D.L.), Lund, Sweden. Sara.Hall@med.lu.se Oskar.Hansson@med.lu.se.
Hansson O	From the Department of Neurology (S.H., Y.S.) and Memory Clinic (O.H.), Skane University Hospital; Department of Clinical Sciences (S.H., Y.S., D.L., O.H.), Lund University; Department of Psychiatry and Neurochemistry (A.O., H.Z.), Institute of Neuroscience and Physiology, the Sahlgrenska Academy at the University of Gothenburg, Gothenburg and Molndal, Sweden; UCL Institute of Neurology (H.Z.), Queen Square, London, UK; and Psychiatry Skane (D.L.), Lund, Sweden. Sara.Hall@med.lu.se Oskar.Hansson@med.lu.se.
Kader M	Department of Health Sciences, Lund University, PO Box 157, SE-221 00, Lund, Sweden. manzur.kader@med.lu.se. Sweden. Hospital, Lund, Sweden. Sweden.
Lindvall O	Laboratory of Stem Cells and Restorative Neurology, Lund Stem Cell Center, University Hospital, Lund, Sweden.

Name of Author	Institutional Affiliation
Nilsson MH	Department of Health Sciences, Lund University, PO Box 157, SE-221 00, Lund, Sweden. manzur.kader@med.lu.se. Sweden. Hospital, Lund, Sweden. Sweden.
Nyholm D	Department of Neuroscience, Neurology, Uppsala University, Uppsala, Sweden.
Parmar M	Department of Experimental Medical Science, Wallenberg Neuroscience Center, Division of Neurobiology and Lund Stem Cell Center, Lund University, BMC A11, S-221 84 Lund, Sweden malin.parmar@med.lu.se.
Senek M	Department of Neuroscience, Neurology, Uppsala University, Uppsala, Sweden.

Switzerland

Name of Author	Institutional Affiliation
Bargiotas P	Department of Neurology, University Hospital (Inselspital) and University of Bern, Bern, Switzerland.; Department of Neurosurgery, University Hospital (Inselspital) and University of Bern, Bern, Switzerland.
Bassetti CL	Department of Neurology, University Hospital (Inselspital) and University of Bern, Bern, Switzerland.; Department of Neurosurgery, University Hospital (Inselspital) and University of Bern, Bern, Switzerland.

Taiwan

Name of Author	Institutional Affiliation
Chiou SM	Department of Neurosurgery, China Medical University Hospital, China Medical University, Taichung, Taiwan. Electronic address: tsmchiou@pchome.com.tw. University, Taichung, Taiwan. University, Taichung, Taiwan.

Name of Author	Institutional Affiliation
Eric Nyam TT	Department of Neurosurgery, Chi Mei Medical Center, Tainan, Taiwan.; Department of Medical Research, Chi Mei Medical Center, Tainan, Taiwan; Department of Hospital and Health Care Administration, Chia Nan University of Pharmacy and Science, Tainan, Taiwan.; Department of Rehabilitation, Chi Mei Medical Center, Tainan, Taiwan.; Department of Neurosurgery, Chi Mei Medical Center, Chiali, Tainan, Taiwan; Department of Nursing, Min-Hwei College of Health Care Management, Tainan, Taiwan.; Department of Medical Research, Chi Mei Medical Center, Tainan, Taiwan.
Huang HM	Department of Neurosurgery, China Medical University Hospital, China Medical University, Taichung, Taiwan. Electronic address: tsmchiou@pchome.com.tw. University, Taichung, Taiwan. University, Taichung, Taiwan.
Jeng C	From the School of Gerontology Health Management, College of Nursing, Taipei Medical University (I-JT); Department of Neurology, Taipei Medical University Hospital (R-YY); and Department of Neurology, School of Medicine, College of Medicine (R-YY), and Graduate Institute of Nursing, College of Nursing (CJ), Taipei Medical University, Taipei, Taiwan.
Liang HW	Department of Physical Medicine and Rehabilitation, National Taiwan University Hospital, Taipei, Taiwan; Department of Physical Medicine and Rehabilitation, National Taiwan University College of Medicine, Taipei, Taiwan. Electronic address: panslcb@gmail.com.; Department of Physical Medicine and Rehabilitation, National Taiwan University Hospital, Yun-Lin Branch, Yunlin, Taiwan.
Lin CH	Section of Neurology, Taichung Veterans General Hospital, Taichung, Taiwan. Taichung, Taiwan.

Name of Author	Institutional Affiliation
Pan SL	Department of Physical Medicine and Rehabilitation, National Taiwan University Hospital, Taipei, Taiwan; Department of Physical Medicine and Rehabilitation, National Taiwan University College of Medicine, Taipei, Taiwan. Electronic address: panslcb@gmail.com.; Department of Physical Medicine and Rehabilitation, National Taiwan University Hospital, Yun-Lin Branch, Yunlin, Taiwan.
Tseng IJ	From the School of Gerontology Health Management, College of Nursing, Taipei Medical University (I-JT); Department of Neurology, Taipei Medical University Hospital (R-YY); and Department of Neurology, School of Medicine, College of Medicine (R-YY), and Graduate Institute of Nursing, College of Nursing (CJ), Taipei Medical University, Taipei, Taiwan.
Wang CC	Department of Neurosurgery, Chi Mei Medical Center, Tainan, Taiwan.; Department of Medical Research, Chi Mei Medical Center, Tainan, Taiwan; Department of Hospital and Health Care Administration, Chia Nan University of Pharmacy and Science, Tainan, Taiwan.; Department of Rehabilitation, Chi Mei Medical Center, Tainan, Taiwan.; Department of Neurosurgery, Chi Mei Medical Center, Chiali, Tainan, Taiwan; Department of Nursing, Min-Hwei College of Health Care Management, Tainan, Taiwan.; Department of Medical Research, Chi Mei Medical Center, Tainan, Taiwan.
Wu YH	Section of Neurology, Taichung Veterans General Hospital, Taichung, Taiwan. Taichung, Taiwan.

United Kingdom

Name of Author	Institutional Affiliation
Aarsland D	KCL-PARCOG Group, Institute of Psychiatry, Psychology and Neuroscience, King's College London, London, UK.; Department of Old Age Psychiatry, Institute of Psychiatry, Psychology and Neuroscience, King's College London, London, UK.; Department of Neurobiology, Care Sciences and Society, Karolinska Institute, Stockholm, Sweden.; University of Exeter Medical School, University of Exeter, Exeter, Devon, UK.; Department of Basic and Clinical Neuroscience, The Maurice Wohl Clinical Neuroscience Institute, King's College London, London, UK.
Alty J	Department of Neurosciences, Leeds Teaching Hospitals NHS Trust, Leeds, West Yorkshire, UK University of Leeds Hull York Medical School, University of York. Yorkshire, UK. Yorkshire, UK. Yorkshire, UK University of Leeds Hull York Medical School, University of York.
Antoniades CA	Nuffield Department of Clinical Neurosciences and chrystalina.antoniades@ndcn.ox.ac.uk james.fitzgerald@nds.ox.ac.uk. United Kingdom. Sciences, University of Oxford, Oxford OX3 9DU, United Kingdom. Sciences, University of Oxford, Oxford OX3 9DU, United Kingdom. Sciences, University of Oxford, Oxford OX3 9DU, United Kingdom chrystalina.antoniades@ndcn.ox.ac.uk james.fitzgerald@nds.ox.ac.uk.
Antonini A	Parkinson and Movement Disorders Unit, IRCCS Hospital San Camillo, Venice, Italy. and Neurosciences, INSERM and Toulouse University Hospital, Toulouse, France. IDIBAPS, Centro de Investigacion Biomedica en Red sobre Enfermedades Neurodegenerativas (CIBERNED), Barcelona Catalonia, Spain. Hospital, Kings College and Kings Health Partners, London, UK.

Name of Author	Institutional Affiliation
Bentivoglio AR	*Sobell Department, UCL Institute of Neurology, Queen Square, London, UK; daggerDepartment of Geriatrics, Neuroscience and Orthopaedics, "Gemelli" Hospital, Catholic University of Sacred Heart (UCSC), Rome; double daggerCattedra di Psichiatria - Dipartimento di Scienze della Salute, Universita` degli Studi di Milano; and section signInstitute of Neurology, Catholic University of Sacred Heart, Rome, Italy.
Bombieri F	Department of Neuroscience, Biomedicine and Movement Sciences, Universita di Verona, Verona, Italy. Verona, Verona, Italy. Verona, Verona, Italy; CeRiSM (Research Centre of Mountain Sport and Health), University of Verona, Rovereto, Italy. Surgery, Neuroscience Section, University of Salerno, Salerno, Italy. Verona, Verona, Italy. Electronic address: michele.tinazzi@univr.it. Surgery, Neuroscience Section, University of Salerno, Salerno, Italy; Sobell Department of Motor Neuroscience and Movement Disorders, University College London (UCL) Institute of Neurology, London, United Kingdom.
Castro Caldas A	a Neurology Service, Department of Neurosciences , Hospital de Santa Maria , Lisbon , Portugal. Portugal. University Hospitals NHS Foundation Trust , London , United Kingdom.
Cavanna AE	1University of Birmingham Medical School,Birmingham,UK. Birmingham,Birmingham,UK. Birmingham,Birmingham,UK.
Chaudhuri KR	a QuintilesIMS , London , UK.

Name of Author	Institutional Affiliation
Erro R	Department of Neuroscience, Biomedicine and Movement Sciences, Universita di Verona, Verona, Italy. Verona, Verona, Italy. Verona, Verona, Italy; CeRiSM (Research Centre of Mountain Sport and Health), University of Verona, Rovereto, Italy. Surgery, Neuroscience Section, University of Salerno, Salerno, Italy. Verona, Verona, Italy. Electronic address: michele.tinazzi@univr.it. Surgery, Neuroscience Section, University of Salerno, Salerno, Italy; Sobell Department of Motor Neuroscience and Movement Disorders, University College London (UCL) Institute of Neurology, London, United Kingdom.
Fasano A	Morton and Gloria Shulman Movement Disorders Centre and the Edmond J. Safra Program in Parkinson's Disease, Toronto Western Hospital, UHN, Division of Neurology, University of Toronto, Toronto, Ontario, Canada. Sydney, Australia. Tel Aviv Sourasky Medical Center, Tel Aviv, Israel. of Medicine, Tel Aviv University, Tel Aviv, Israel. University Medical Center, Chicago, Illinois, US. Newcastle upon Tyne, UK.
Ferreira JJ	a Neurology Service, Department of Neurosciences , Hospital de Santa Maria , Lisbon , Portugal. Portugal. University Hospitals NHS Foundation Trust , London , United Kingdom.
Ffytche DH	KCL-PARCOG Group, Institute of Psychiatry, Psychology and Neuroscience, King's College London, London, UK.; Department of Old Age Psychiatry, Institute of Psychiatry, Psychology and Neuroscience, King's College London, London, UK.; Department of Neurobiology, Care Sciences and Society, Karolinska Institute, Stockholm, Sweden.; University of Exeter Medical School, University of Exeter, Exeter, Devon, UK.; Department of Basic and Clinical Neuroscience, The Maurice Wohl Clinical Neuroscience Institute, King's College London, London, UK.

Name of Author	Institutional Affiliation
FitzGerald JJ	Nuffield Department of Clinical Neurosciences and chrystalina.antoniades@ndcn.ox.ac.uk james.fitzgerald@nds.ox.ac.uk. United Kingdom. Sciences, University of Oxford, Oxford OX3 9DU, United Kingdom. Sciences, University of Oxford, Oxford OX3 9DU, United Kingdom. Sciences, University of Oxford, Oxford OX3 9DU, United Kingdom chrystalina.antoniades@ndcn.ox.ac.uk james.fitzgerald@nds.ox.ac.uk.
Goedert M	Laboratory of Molecular Biology, Medical Research Council, Francis Crick Avenue, Cambridge CB2 0QH, UK. mg@mrc-lmb.cam.ac.uk.
Hindle Fisher I	1University of Birmingham Medical School,Birmingham,UK. Birmingham,Birmingham,UK. Birmingham,Birmingham,UK.
Jamieson S	Department of Neurosciences, Leeds Teaching Hospitals NHS Trust, Leeds, West Yorkshire, UK University of Leeds Hull York Medical School, University of York. Yorkshire, UK. Yorkshire, UK. Yorkshire, UK University of Leeds Hull York Medical School, University of York.
Jenner P	Department of Clinical Neurosciences, University College London (UCL) Institute of Neurology, Royal Free Campus, Rowland Hill Street, London NW3 2PF, UK. Hospital, King's College London, Camberwell Road, London SE5 9RS, UK. Faculty of Life Sciences and Medicine, King's College London, Newcomen Street, London SE1 1UL, UK.
Karabiyik C	Department of Medical Genetics, Cambridge Institute for Medical Research, Cambridge Biomedical Campus, Wellcome Trust/MRC Building, Cambridge Biomedical Campus, Hills Road, Cambridge CB2 0XY, U.K. College of Medicine, Seoul 03080, Korea dcr1000@cam.ac.uk minjlee@snu.ac.kr. Cambridge Biomedical Campus, Wellcome Trust/MRC Building, Cambridge Biomedical Campus, Hills Road, Cambridge CB2 0XY, U.K. dcr1000@cam.ac.uk minjlee@snu.ac.kr. Campus, Hills Road, Cambridge, U.K.

Name of Author	Institutional Affiliation
Lord S	Human Movement Science, Institute of Neuroscience, Newcastle University Institute for Aging, Newcastle University, Newcastle upon Tyne, NE4 5PL, UK. lynn.rochester@ncl.ac.uk.; NIHR Newcastle Biomedical Research Centre, Newcastle upon Tyne Hospitals NHS Foundation Trust and Newcastle University, Newcastle upon Tyne, UK. lynn.rochester@ncl.ac.uk.; School of Clinical Sciences, Auckland University of Technology, Auckland, New Zealand.; Newcastle upon Tyne Hospitals NHS Foundation Trust, Newcastle upon Tyne, UK. lynn.rochester@ncl.ac.uk.; UK and Industrial Statistics Research Unit, Newcastle University, Newcastle upon Tyne, UK.
Lowin J	a QuintilesIMS , London , UK.
Ray Chaudhuri K	a Department of Neurology, Neurosurgery and Medical Genetics, Federal State Budgetary Educational Institution of Higher Education , 'N.I. Pirogov Russian National Research Medical University' of the Ministry of Healthcare of the Russian Federation , Moscow , Russia. Excellence , Kings College and Kings College Hospital , London , UK. London , UK.
Ricciardi L	*Sobell Department, UCL Institute of Neurology, Queen Square, London, UK; daggerDepartment of Geriatrics, Neuroscience and Orthopaedics, "Gemelli" Hospital, Catholic University of Sacred Heart (UCSC), Rome; double daggerCattedra di Psichiatria - Dipartimento di Scienze della Salute, Universita` degli Studi di Milano; and section signInstitute of Neurology, Catholic University of Sacred Heart, Rome, Italy.

Name of Author	Institutional Affiliation
Rochester L	Human Movement Science, Institute of Neuroscience, Newcastle University Institute for Aging, Newcastle University, Newcastle upon Tyne, NE4 5PL, UK. lynn.rochester@ncl.ac.uk.; NIHR Newcastle Biomedical Research Centre, Newcastle upon Tyne Hospitals NHS Foundation Trust and Newcastle University, Newcastle upon Tyne, UK. lynn.rochester@ncl.ac.uk.; School of Clinical Sciences, Auckland University of Technology, Auckland, New Zealand.; Newcastle upon Tyne Hospitals NHS Foundation Trust, Newcastle upon Tyne, UK. lynn.rochester@ncl.ac.uk.; UK and Industrial Statistics Research Unit, Newcastle University, Newcastle upon Tyne, UK.
Rubinsztein DC	Department of Medical Genetics, Cambridge Institute for Medical Research, Cambridge Biomedical Campus, Wellcome Trust/MRC Building, Cambridge Biomedical Campus, Hills Road, Cambridge CB2 0XY, U.K. College of Medicine, Seoul 03080, Korea dcr1000@cam.ac.uk minjlee@snu.ac.kr. Cambridge Biomedical Campus, Wellcome Trust/MRC Building, Cambridge Biomedical Campus, Hills Road, Cambridge CB2 0XY, U.K. dcr1000@cam.ac.uk minjlee@snu.ac.kr. Campus, Hills Road, Cambridge, U.K.
Schapira A	a Department of Clinical Neurosciences , Institute of Neurology, University College London , London , UK. College London , London , UK.
Schapira AHV	Department of Clinical Neurosciences, University College London (UCL) Institute of Neurology, Royal Free Campus, Rowland Hill Street, London NW3 2PF, UK. Hospital, King's College London, Camberwell Road, London SE5 9RS, UK. Faculty of Life Sciences and Medicine, King's College London, Newcomen Street, London SE1 1UL, UK.

Name of Author	Institutional Affiliation
Titova N	a Department of Neurology, Neurosurgery and Medical Genetics, Federal State Budgetary Educational Institution of Higher Education , 'N.I. Pirogov Russian National Research Medical University' of the Ministry of Healthcare of the Russian Federation , Moscow , Russia. Excellence , Kings College and Kings College Hospital , London , UK. London , UK.
deSouza RM	a Department of Clinical Neurosciences , Institute of Neurology, University College London , London , UK. College London , London , UK.

NOTES

Use this page for taking notes as you review your Guidebook

5 - Tips on Finding and Choosing a Doctor

Introduction

One of the most important decisions confronting patients who have been diagnosed with a serious medical condition is finding and choosing a qualified physician who will deliver a high level and quality of medical care in accordance with currently accepted guidelines and standards of care. Finding the "best" doctor to manage your condition, however, can be a frustrating and time-consuming experience unless you know what you are looking for and how to go about finding it.

The process of finding and choosing a physician to manage your specific illness or condition is, in some respects, analogous to the process of making a decision about whether or not to invest in a particular stock or mutual fund. After all, you wouldn't invest your hard eared money in a stock or mutual fund without first doing exhaustive research about the stock or fund's past performance, current financial status, and projected future earnings. More than likely you would spend a considerable amount of time and energy doing your own research and consulting with your stock broker before making an informed decision about investing. The same general principle applies to the process of finding and choosing a physician. Although the process requires a considerable investment in terms of both time and energy, the potential payoff can be well worth it--after all, what can be more important than your health and well-being?

This section of your Guidebook offers important tips for how to find physicians as well as suggestions for how to make informed choices about choosing a doctor who is right for you.

Tips for Finding Physicians

Finding a highly qualified, competent, and compassionate physician to manage your specific illness or condition takes a lot of hard work and energy but is an investment that is well-worth the effort. It is important to keep in mind that you are not looking for just any general physician but rather for a physician who has expertise in the treatment and management of your specific illness or condition. Here are some suggestions for where you can turn to identify and locate physicians who specialize in managing your disorder:

- **Your Doctor** - Your family physician (family medicine or internal medicine specialist) is a good starting point for finding a physician who specializes in your illness. Chances are that your doctor already knows several specialists in your geographic area who specialize in your illness and can recommend several names to you. Your doctor can also provide you with information about their qualifications, training, and hospital affiliations.

- **Your Peer Network** - Your family, friends, and co-workers can be a potentially very useful network for helping you find a physician who specializes in your illness. They may know someone else with this condition and may be able to put you in touch with them to find out which doctors they can recommend. If you have friends, neighbors, or relatives who work in hospitals (e.g., nurses, social workers, administrators), they may be a potentially valuable source for helping you find a physician who specializes in your condition.

- **Hospitals and Medical Centers** - Hospitals and medical centers are, potentially, an excellent source for finding physicians who specialize in treating specific diseases. Simply contact hospitals and major medical centers in your city, county, or state and ask if they have anyone on their staff who specializes in treating your condition. When you call, ask to speak to someone in the specific Department that cares for patients with the illness. For example, if you have been diagnosed with cancer, ask to speak with someone in the Department of Hematology and Oncology. If you are not sure which Department treats patients with your specific condition, ask to speak to someone in the Department of Medicine since this Department is the umbrella for many other medical specialties.

- **Organizations and Support Groups** - Many disease organizations and support groups that cater to patients with a specific illness or condition maintain physician referral lists and may be able to recommend doctors in your geographic area who specialize in the treatment and management of your specific disorder. This *MediFocus Guidebook* includes a select listing of disease organizations and support groups that you may wish to contact to ask for a physician referral.

- **Managed Care Plans** - If you belong to a managed care plan, you can obtain a list of physicians who belong to the Plan from the plan's membership services office. Keep in mind, however, that your choices will usually be limited to only those doctors who belong to the Plan. If you decide to go outside the Plan, you will likely have to pay for the doctor's services "out of pocket".

- **Medical Journals** - Many doctors based at major medical centers and universities who have special interest in a particular disease or condition conduct research and publish their findings in leading medical journals. Searching the medical literature can help you identify and locate leading physicians who are recognized as experts in their field about a particular illness. This *MediFocus Guidebook* includes an extensive listing of the names and institutional affiliations of physicians and researchers, in the United States and other countries, who have recently published their studies about this specific medical condition in leading medical journals. You can also conduct your own online search for your illness or condition and identify additional authors and hospitals who specialize in the disease using the PubMed database available at http://www.nlm.nih.gov.

- **American Medical Association** - The American Medical Association (AMA) is the nation's largest professional medical association that represents many doctors in the United States and also provides a free physician locator service called "AMA Physician Select" available at http://dbapps.ama-assn.org/aps/amahg.htm. You can search the AMA database by either "Physician Name" or "Medical Specialty". You can find information about physicians including medical school and residency training, area of specialty, and contact information.

- **American Board of Medical Specialists** - The American Board of Medical Specialists (ABMS) publishes a geographical list of board-certified physicians called the Official ABMS Directory of Board Certified Medical Specialists that is available in most public libraries. Physicians who are listed in the ABMS Directory are board-certified in a medical specialty meaning that they have passed rigorous certification examinations administered by a board of medical specialists. There are 24 specialty boards that are recognized by the ABMS and the AMA. Each candidate applying for board certification must pass a written examination given by the specific specialty board and 15 of the specialty boards also require candidates to pass an oral examination in order to obtain board certification. To find out if a particular physician you are considering is board certified:

    - Visit your local public library and ask for a copy of the Official ABMS Directory of Board Certified Medical Specialists.

    - Search the ABMS web site at http://www.abms.org/login.asp.

    - Call the ABMS toll free at 1-866-275-2267.

- **American Society of Clinical Oncology** - The American Society of Clinical Onclology (ASC)) is the largest professional organization that represents physicians who specialize in treating cancer patients (oncologists). The ASCO provides a searchable database of ASCO members called "Find an Oncologist" that you can access online at http://www.asco.org. You can search the "Find an Oncologist" database for a cancer specialist by name, city, state, country, or specialty area.

- **American Cancer Society** - The American Cancer Society (ACS) is a nationwide voluntary health organization dedicated to helping cancer patients and survivors through research, education, advocacy, and services. The ACS web site http://www.cancer.org is not only an excellent resource for cancer information but also includes a "Message Board" where you can ask questions, exchange ideas, and share stories. The ACS Message Board is also a potentially useful source for locating an oncologist in your geographical area who specializes in your specific type of cancer. You can also contact the ACS toll free by calling 1-800-ACS-2345.

- **National Comprehensive Cancer Network** - The National Comprehensive Cancer Network (NCCN) is an alliance of 19 of the world's leading cancer centers and is dedicated to helping patients and health care professionals make informed decisions about cancer care. You can find a listing of the 19 NCCN member cancer institutions on the NCCN web site at http://www.nccn.org/. You can also search the NCCN "Physician Directory" for doctors located at any of the 19 NCCN member cancer institutions at http://www.nccn.org/physician_directory/SearchPers.asp. This database is an excellent resource for locating leading cancer specialists nationwide who specialize in your specific type of cancer.

- **National Cancer Institute Clinical Trials Database** - The National Cancer Institute (NCI) is part of the National Institutes of Health (NIH) and coordinates the National Cancer Program which conducts and supports research, training, and a variety of other programs dedicated to prevention and treatment of cancer. The NCI maintains an extensive cancer clinical trials database that you can access at http://www.cancer.gov/clinicaltrials. You can search the database for current clinical trials by type of cancer and even limit your search to clinical trials within you geographical area by putting in your Zip Code. The NCI clinical trials database also provides contact information for the physicians who serve as the study coordinators for each clinical trial. This database is a valuable resource for identifying and locating leading physicians in your local area and around the country who are conducting cutting-edge clinical research about your specific type of cancer.

- **National Center for Complementary and Alternative Medicine** - The National Center for Complementary and Alternative Medicine (NCCAM) is part of the National Institutes of Health (NIH) and is dedicated to exploring complementary and alternative medicine healing practices in the context of rigorous scientific research and methodology. The NCCAM web site http://nccam.nih.gov/ includes publications, frequently asked questions, and useful links to other complementary and alternative medicine resources. If you have questions about complementary and alternative medicine practices for your particular illness or medical condition, you can contact the NCCAM Clearinghouse toll-free in the U.S. at 1-888-644-6226 or 301-519-3153. You can also contact the NCCAM Clearinghouse by E-mail: info@nccam.nih.gov.

- **National Organization for Rare Disorders** - The National Organization for Rare Disorders (NORD) is a federation of voluntary health organizations dedicated to helping patients with rare "orphan" diseases and their families. There are over 6,000 rare or "orphan" diseases that are estimated to affect approximately 25 million Americans. You can search NORD's "Rare Diseases Database" for information about rare diseases at http://www.rarediseases.org/search/rdblist.html. In addition to providing useful information about rare diseases, NORD maintains a confidential "Networking Program" for its members to enable them to communicate with other patients who suffer from the same disorder. To learn more about NORD's Networking Program, you can send an E mail to: orphan@rarediseases.org.

How to Make Informed Choices About Physicians

It has generally been assumed by many people that the longer a physician has been in practice, the more experience, knowledge, and skills he/she has accumulated and, therefore, the higher the quality of care they provide to their patients. Recent research conducted by a group of doctors from the Harvard Medical School, however, seems to strongly suggest that this premise may not be true. In an article published in February 2005 in the *Annals of Internal Medicine* (Volume 142, No. 4, pp. 260-303), the Harvard researchers seriously challenged the common assumption that the more clinical experience a physician has accumulated, the higher the level of medical care they provide to their patients.

In fact, surprisingly, the researchers found an inverse (opposite) relationship between the number of years that a physician has been in practice (i.e., experience) and the quality of care that the physician provides. In other words, the widely held belief that "practice makes perfect" does not necessarily apply to all physicians and should not be the sole criteria used by patients in their decision analysis for choosing a physician. The underlying message of this study is that the length of time a physician has been in practice does not necessarily equate to a high quality of medical care unless the doctor takes steps to keep abreast with new advances and changing patterns of clinical practice.

Here are some important issues you need to consider and carefully research before making an informed decision about choosing your doctor:

- **Board Certification** - Board certified doctors are required to have extra training after medical school to become specialists in a particular field of medicine and are required to take continuing education courses in order to maintain their board certification status. Check with the American Board of Medical Specialists (ABMS) to determine if a specific physician you are considering is board certified in a particular medical specialty. To find out if a particular physician you are considering is board certified:

    - Visit your local public library and ask for a copy of the Official ABMS Directory of Board Certified Medical Specialists.

    - Search the ABMS web site at http://www.abms.org/login.asp.

    - Call the ABMS toll free at 1-866-275-2267.

- **Experience** - As noted above, research from the Harvard Medical School strongly suggests that how long a physician has been in practice (i.e., experience) does not necessarily correlate with a high level of medical care. The most important issue, therefore, is not how long a doctor has been in practice but rather how much experience the physician has in treating your specific illness or medical condition. Some physicians who have been in practice for many decades may have only treated a small number of patients with the specific disorder, whereas, some younger physicians who have been in practice only a few years may have already treated hundreds of patients with the same disorder. Here are some suggestions for helping you find out about a particular physician's experience in treating your specific illness:

    - Call the physician's office and speak with a staff member such as a nurse or physician's assistant. Ask them for information about how many patients with your specific medical condition the physician treats during the course of a year. Ask how many patients with this condition the physician is currently treating. You will have to call several different physicians' offices in order to have a basis for comparing the numbers of patients.

    - Find out if the physician has published any articles about the condition in reputable medical journals by doing an author search online. You can conduct an online author search using PubMed at http://www.nlm.nih.gov. Simply click on the "PubMed" icon, select the "author" field from the "Limits" menu, enter the physician's name (last name followed by first initial), and then click on the "Go" button. The author search will retrieve all articles published by the particular physician you are considering.

- Talk with your family physician and ask if he/she can provide you with any information about the particular physician's experience in treating patients with your specific illness or condition.

- Contact disease organizations and support groups that specialize in helping patients with your specific disorder and ask if they can provide you with any information, including experience, about the physician you are considering.

- **Medical School Affiliation** - Find out if the physician you are considering also has a joint faculty appointment at a medical school. In general, practicing community physicians with a joint academic appointment at a medical school are more likely to be in contact with leading medical experts and may be more up-to-date with the latest advances in research and treatments than community based physicians who are not affiliated with a medical school.

- **Hospital Affiliation** - Find out about the hospitals that the doctor uses. In the event that you need to be treated at a hospital, is the hospital where the physician has admitting privileges nearby to your home or will you (and your family members) have to travel a considerable distance?

- **Hospital Accreditation** - Find out if the hospital where the physician has admitting privileges is accredited by the Joint Commission on Accreditation of Healthcare Organizations (JCAHO). You can find information about a specific hospital's accreditation status by searching the JCAHO web site at http://www.jointcommission.org/. The JCAHO is an independent, not-for-profit organization that evaluates and accredits more than 15,000 health care organizations and programs in the United States. To receive and maintain JCAHO accreditation, a health care organization must undergo an on-site survey by a JCAHO survey team at least every three years and meet specific standards and performance measurements that affect the safety and quality of patient care.

- **Health Insurance Coverage** - Find out if the physician is covered by your health insurance plan. If you belong to a managed care plan (HMO or PPO), you are usually restricted to using specific physicians who also belong to the Plan. If you decide to use a physician who is "outside the network," you will likely have to pay "out of pocket" for the services provided.

NOTES

Use this page for taking notes as you review your Guidebook

6 - Directory of Organizations

American Academy of Neurology

201 Chicago Avenue, Minneapolis, MN 55415
800.879.1960
memberservies@aan.com
www.aan.com

American Association of Neurological Surgeons

5550 Meadowbrook Drive, Rolling Meadows, IL 60088
888.566.AANS 847.378-0500
info@aans.org
www.aans.org

American Parkinson Disease Association

135 Parkinson Avenue; Staten Island, NY 10305
718.981.8001; 800.223.2732
apda@apdaparkinson.org
www.apdaparkinson.org

APDA National Young Onset Center

63 West Main St, Suite H, Freehold, NJ 07728
800- 838-0879
www.wellspouse.org

Bachmann-Strauss Dystonia & Parkinsons Disease Foundation

Mt. Sinai Medical Center; Fred French Building 551 5th Avenue Suite 520 New York, NY 10176
212.682.9900
www.dystonia-parkinsons.org

Cargiver Action Network

1150 Connecticut Avenue; #501; Kensington, MD 20036-3904
202-454-3970
info@caregiveraction.org
www.caregiveraction.org/

Daily Strength's PD Support Group

https://www.dailystrength.org/group/parkinson-s-disease

DBSsurgery Yahoo! Group

https://groups.yahoo.com/neo/groups/DBSsurgery/info

European Parkinsons Disease Association

1 Cobden Road, Sevenoaks, Kent, TN13 3UB, United Kingdom
info@epda.eu.com
www.epda.eu.com

Family Caregiver Alliance

235 Montgomery Street; Suite 950; San Francisco, CA 94104
800.445.8106 415.434.3388
info@caregiver.org
www.caregiver.org

International Parkinson and Movement Disorder Society

555 East Wells Street; Suite 1100; Milwaukee, WI 53202-3823
414.276.2145
info@movementdisorders.org
www.movementdisorders.org

Michael J. Fox Foundation for Parkinson's Research

Grand Central Station, P.O. Box 4777 New York, NY 10163-4777
800.708.7644
michaeljfox.org

Parkinson Canada

4211 Yonge Street; Suite 316; Toronto, M2P 2A9 CANADA
800.565.3000 416.227.9700
info@parkinson.ca
www.parkinson.ca

Parkinson's Foundation

1359 Broadway; Suite 1509; New York, NY 10018
800.473.4636
helpline@parkinson.org
www.pdf.org

Parkinson's Foundation Open Forum

forum.parkinson.org/forum/3-open-forum/

Parkinson's UK

215 Vauxhall Bridge Road; London SW1V 1EJ; UNITED KINGDOM
Phone: 0808 800 0303 ; Text relay: 18001 0808 800 0303
hello@parkinsons.org.uk
www.parkinsons.org.uk

Parkinson's Resource Organization

74090 El Passeo; Suite 102; Palm Desert, CA 92260-4135
877.775.4111; 760.773.5628
info@parkinsonsresource.org
www.parkinsonsresource.org

Parkinson's Australia

PO Box 108, Deakin West, ACT 2600
0407 703 328
info@parkinsons.org.au
www.parkinsons.org.au

PatientsLikeMe Forum

https://www.patientslikeme.com/

Smart Patients Parkinson's Disease Community

https://www.smartpatients.com/partners/apda

The Cure Parkinson's Trust

120 Baker Street, London W1U 6TU, United Kingdom
020 7487 3892
cptinfo@cureparkinsons.org.uk
www.cureparkinsons.org.uk

The Parkinson Alliance

POB 308; Kingston, NJ 08528
800.579.8440 609.688.0870
www.parkinsonalliance.org

The Parkinson's Institute and Clinical Center

675 Almanor Avenue Sunnyvale, CA 94085
800.655.2273 408.734.2800
www.thepi.org

Complementary and Alternative Medicine Resources

American Academy of Medical Acupuncture

170 East Grand Avenue Suite 330 El Segundo, CA 90245 Phone: 310.364.0193
administrato@medicalacupuncture.org
http://www.medicalacupuncture.org

American Association for Acupuncture and Oriental Medicine

1925 West County Road B2
Roseville, MN 55113
Phone: 651.631.0216
http://www.aaaom.edu

American Association of Naturopathic Physicians

4435 Wisconsin Avenue
Suite 403 Washington, DC 20016
Phone (Toll free): 866.538.2267
Phone: 202.237.8150
http://www.naturopathic.org

American Chiropractic Association

1701 Clarendon Blvd.
Arlington, VA 22209
Phone: 703.276.8800 memberinfo@acatoday.org http://www.amerchiro.org

American Holistic Medical Association

23366 Commerce Park Suite 101B Beachwood, OH 44122 Phone: 216.292.6644
info@holisticmedicine.org http://www.holisticmedicine.org

American Massage Therapy Association

500 Davis Street, Suite 900
Evanston, IL 60201-4695
Phone (Toll-Free): 877.905.2700
Phone: 847.864.0123 info@amtamassage.org http://www.amtamassage.org

National Center for Complementary and Alternative Medicine (NCCAM) Clearinghouse

9000 Rockville Pike Bethesda, MD 20892 Phone: 888.644.6226 info@nccam.nih.gov http://nccam.nih.gov

National Center for Homeopathy

801 North Fairfax Street, Suite 306
Alexandria, VA 22314
Phone: 703.548.7790
http://www.homeopathic.org

Office of Dietary Supplements, National Institutes of Health

6100 Executive Boulevard
Room 3B01, MSC 7517
Bethesda, MD 20892-7517
Phone: 301.435.2920 ods@nih.gov http://ods.od.nih.gov

Rosenthal Center for Complementary and Alternative Medicine

Columbia Presbyterian Hospital
630 West 168th Street
Box 75
New York, NY 10032
Phone: 212.342.0101
http://rosenthal.hs.columbia.edu

CPSIA information can be obtained
at www.ICGtesting.com
Printed in the USA
BVHW010222250121
598665BV00020B/774